The Vegan Bod Cookbo

CW01456308

101 Plant-Based, High-Protein, Low-Carb Recipes to Fuel Your High-Performance Muscle Mass Building. Bulk Up Naturally Without Giving Up Your Health and Principles

SCOTT NARDELLA

© Copyright 2020 by *Scott Nardella*

All rights reserved.

This document is geared towards providing exact and reliable information with regards to the topic and issue covered. The publication is sold with the idea that the publisher is not required to render accounting, officially permitted, or otherwise, qualified services. If advice is necessary, legal or professional, a practiced individual in the profession should be ordered.

- From a Declaration of Principles which was accepted and approved equally by a Committee of the American Bar Association and a Committee of Publishers and Associations.

In no way is it legal to reproduce, duplicate, or transmit any part of this document in either electronic means or in printed format. Recording of this publication is strictly prohibited and any storage of this document is not allowed unless with written permission from the publisher. All rights reserved.

The information provided herein is stated to be truthful and consistent, in that any liability, in terms of inattention or otherwise, by any usage or abuse of any policies, processes, or directions contained within is the solitary and utter responsibility of the recipient reader. Under no circumstances will any legal responsibility or blame be held against the publisher for any reparation, damages, or monetary loss due to the information herein, either directly or indirectly.

Respective authors own all copyrights not held by the publisher.

The information herein is offered for informational purposes solely, and is universal as so. The presentation of the information is without contract or any type of guarantee assurance.

The trademarks that are used are without any consent, and the publication of the trademark is without permission or backing by the trademark owner. All trademarks and brands within this book are for clarifying purposes only and are the owned by the owners themselves, not affiliated with this document

Table of Contents

INTRODUCTION

After I wrote my book "The Vegan Bodybuilder" I received a lot of compliments by bodybuilders, and athletes in general, to be honest, telling me how great it was for them to have so useful information delivered in a very clear way, to back them up in this not always easy pathway of balancing an intense athletic life and a plant based diet.

Bodybuilder and vegan. Two ways of life that are challenging in themselves, let alone combined.

Bodybuilder and Vegan.

Even without considering that you have to deal with all these people explaining you that you can't do that, and why you can't, and why eating animals is your real nature, and why to build muscle you need animal proteins, and the entire repertoire of common myths and misconceptions, even all this aside, being a vegan and a bodybuilder is still not a walk in the park.

Being a bodybuilder, or an athlete in general, requires a lot of discipline, focus, sacrifice. You may need to wake up very early to train before you go to work, you may spend the evening under the bar instead than at the bar, and you have to be careful of your diet too.

Being a vegan may mean sacrifice too, if you are not lucky enough to just dislike meat or animal products. After all these years I don't miss these kinds of meals at all , but I know many people that gave up meat "just" because this felt right to them, in spite of how they loved it. I respect them infinitely for keeping on vegan while missing animal food every day.

But even if you are a "natural" vegan, and you don't suffer at all the giving up, there is no shortage of difficulties. You end soon get used to that, but, even if it's objectively easier than 15 or 20 years ago, if you shop in non specialized stores you often have to check for hidden animal byproducts written in very small letters on the label, like animal fats in industrial bakery products, and there are still restaurants that can't offer a real vegan alternative other than a salad (and sometimes they still ask you if you are ok with some eggs and cheese in it).

So in this scenario I received many messages of people thanking me for having helped them keeping these two challenges together.

And this was, of course, my greatest satisfaction. I am absolutely honest when I say that I didn't received any negative feedback (I'm not on facebook, this helped for sure), but since I'm always looking for what I could have done better, I have noticed that many readers told me things like "this is great, sadly it is just not easy to have always new ideas for recipes that fit this lifestyle" or "too bad that most of the vegan cookbooks out there are meant for a classic balanced diet or for weight loss, and not for high protein as we need" or simply "I loved the book, can you suggest me some recipe?".

And this is why, after some recipes sent by email to people that asked me, I decided to write this book with no theory (you know it all from The Vegan Bodybuilder already!) and just recipes.

There are 101 of them, and an example of a 4 weeks meal plan too. I really hope you enjoy it, and please feel free to let me know if there's something I could have done better, that there always is, as we perfectly know.

You can write to me at zhnardella@gmail.com, I would really appreciate both compliments and suggestions, and I usually answer to everyone (maybe not immediately, but I will).

Enjoy!

P.S. I gave some of the recipes bodybuilding related names, this is just for fun, you don't need to have Pushups Muffins to do push ups or Leg Day Pancakes on your leg day (even though... why not?)

BREAKFASTS

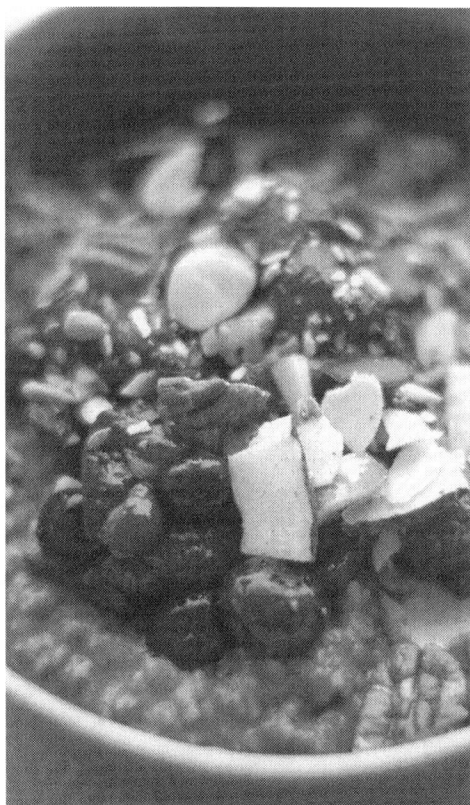

Breakfast is the most important meal of the day.

To be honest, this is not always true, but generally speaking, if you face your energy demanding day with the right fueling of nutrients you are starting off on the right foot.

01. FRUIT GRANOLA

Preparation time: 15 min
Cook time: 45 min
Total time: 60 min
Serves: 5

Ingredients

2 cups rolled oats
¾ cup whole-grain flour
1 tablespoon ground cinnamon
1 teaspoon ground ginger (optional)
½ cup sunflower seeds, or walnuts, chopped
½ cup almonds, chopped

½ cup pumpkin seeds
½ cup unsweetened shredded coconut
1¼ cups pure fruit juice (cranberry, apple or similar)
½ cup raisins, or dried cranberries
½ cup goji berries (optional)

Preparation

Preheat the oven to 350°F.

Mix together the oats, flour, cinnamon, ginger, sunflower seeds, almonds, pumpkin seeds, and coconut in a large bowl.

Sprinkle the juice over the mixture, and stir until it's just moistened. You might need a bit more or a bit less liquid, depending on how much your oats and flour absorb.

Spread the granola on a large baking sheet (the more spread out it is the better), and put it in the oven. After about 15 minutes, use a spatula to turn the granola so that the middle gets dried out. Let the granola bake until it's as crunchy as you want it, about 30 minutes more.

Take the granola out of the oven and stir in the raisins and goji berries (if using). Store leftovers in an airtight container for up to 2 weeks.

Serve with non-dairy milk and fresh fruit, use as a topper for morning porridge or a smoothie bowl to add a bit of crunch, or make a granola parfait by layering with non-dairy yogurt or puréed banana.

Per Serving (½ cup) Calories: 398; Protein: 11g; Total fat: 25g; Carbohydrates: 39g; Fiber: 8g

02. PUMPKIN STEEL-CUT OATS

Preparation time: 2 min
Cook time: 35 min
Total time:37 min
Serves: 4

Ingredients

3 cups water

1 cup steel-cut oats

½ cup canned pumpkin purée

¼ cup pumpkin seeds (pepitas)

2 tablespoons maple syrup

Pinch salt

Preparation

In a large saucepan, bring the water to a boil.

Add the oats, stir, and reduce the heat to low. Simmer until the oats are soft, 20 to 30 minutes, continuing to stir occasionally.

Stir in the pumpkin purée and continue cooking on low for 3 to 5 minutes longer. Stir in the pumpkin seeds and maple syrup, and season with the salt.

Divide the oatmeal into 4 single-serving containers. Let cool before sealing the lids.

Place the containers in the refrigerator for up to 5 days.

Per Serving: Calories:121; Protein: 4g; Total fat: 5g; Carbohydrates: 17g; Fiber: 2g

03. Choco-Quinoa Energy Bowl

Preparation time: 5 min
Cook time: 30 min
Total time: 35 min
Serves: 2

Ingredients

2 to 3 tablespoons unsweetened cocoa powder, or carob
1 to 2 tablespoons almond butter, or other nut or seed butter
1 tablespoon ground flaxseed, or chia or hemp seeds
2 tablespoons walnuts
¼ cup raspberries

1 cup quinoa
1 teaspoon ground cinnamon
1 cup non-dairy milk
1 cup water
1 large banana

Preparation

Preparing the Ingredients.

Put the quinoa, cinnamon, milk, and water in a medium pot. Bring to a boil over high heat, then turn down low and simmer, covered, for 25 to 30 minutes.

While the quinoa is simmering, purée or mash the banana in a medium bowl and stir in the cocoa powder, almond butter, and flaxseed.

To serve, spoon 1 cup cooked quinoa into a bowl, top with half the pudding and half the walnuts and raspberries.

Per Serving: Calories: 392; Protein: 12g; Total fat: 19g; Saturated fat: 1g; Carbohydrates: 49g; Fiber: 10g

04. MUESLIBERRY BREAKFAST

Prep: 10 min
Cook Time: 0 min
Total: 10 min
Serves: 5

Ingredients

For The Muesli

1 cup rolled oats
1 cup spelt flakes, or quinoa flakes, or more rolled oats
2 cups puffed cereal
¼ cup sunflower seeds
¼ cup almonds

¼ cup raisins
¼ cup dried cranberries
¼ cup chopped dried figs
¼ cup unsweetened shredded coconut
¼ cup non-dairy chocolate chips
1 to 3 teaspoons ground cinnamon

For The Bowl

1 cup non-dairy milk, or unsweetened applesauce
¾ cup muesli
½ cup berries

Preparation

Preparing the Ingredients.

Put the muesli ingredients in a container or bag and shake.

Combine the muesli and bowl ingredients in a bowl or to-go container.

Substitutions: Try chopped Brazil nuts, peanuts, dried cranberries, dried blueberries, dried mango, or whatever inspires you. Ginger and cardamom are interesting flavors if you want to branch out on spices.

Per Serving: Calories: 441; Protein: 10g; Total fat: 20g; Carbohydrates: 63g; Fiber: 13g.

05. CINNASPICY OATS

Prep: 10 Minutes
Overnight To Soak
Serves: 5

Ingredients

2 ½ cups old-fashioned rolled oats

5 tablespoons pumpkin seeds (pepitas)

5 tablespoons chopped pecans

5 cups unsweetened plant-based milk

2½ teaspoons maple syrup or agave syrup

½ to 1 teaspoon salt

½ to 1 teaspoon ground cinnamon

½ to 1 teaspoon ground ginger

Fresh fruit (optional)

Preparation

Preparing the Ingredients.

Line up 5 wide-mouth pint jars. In each jar, combine ½ cup of oats, 1 tablespoon of pumpkin seeds, 1 tablespoon of pecans, 1 cup of plant-based milk, ½ teaspoon of maple syrup, 1 pinch of salt, 1 pinch of cinnamon, and 1 pinch of ginger.

Stir the ingredients in each jar. Close the jars tightly with lids. To serve, top with fresh fruit (if using). Place the airtight jars in the refrigerator at least overnight before eating and for up to 5 days.

Per Serving: Calories:177; Protein: 6g; Total fat: 9g; Carbohydrates: 19g; Fiber: 4g.

06. FRENCH BANANA TOAST

Prep: 10 Minutes
Cook Time: 30 Minutes
Total: 40 Minutes
Serves: 8 Slices

Ingredients

For The French Toast

1 banana
1 cup coconut milk
1 teaspoon pure vanilla extract
¼ teaspoon ground nutmeg

½ teaspoon ground cinnamon
1½ teaspoons arrowroot powder
Pinch sea salt
8 slices whole-grain bread

For The Raspberry Syrup

1 cup fresh or frozen raspberries, or other berries
2 tablespoons water, or pure fruit juice
1 to 2 tablespoons maple syrup, or coconut sugar (optional)

Preparation

Preparing the Ingredients.

Preheat the oven to 350°F.

In a shallow bowl, purée or mash the banana well. Mix in the coconut milk, vanilla, nutmeg, cinnamon, arrowroot, and salt.

Dip the slices of bread in the banana mixture, and then lay them out in a 13-by-9-inch baking dish.

They should cover the bottom of the dish and can overlap a bit but shouldn't be stacked on top of each other. Pour any leftover banana mixture over the bread, and put the dish in the oven.

Bake for about 30 minutes, or until the tops are lightly browned.

Serve topped with raspberry syrup.

To Make The Raspberry Syrup:

Heat the raspberries in a small pot with the water and the maple syrup (if using) on medium heat.

Leave to simmer, stirring occasionally and breaking up the berries, for 15 to 20 minutes, until the liquid has reduced.

Leftover raspberry syrup makes a great topping for simple oatmeal as a quick and delicious breakfast, or as a drizzle on top of whole-grain toast smeared with natural peanut butter.

Per Serving: Calories: 166; Protein: 5g; Total fat: 7g; Saturated fat: 1g; Carbohydrates: 23g;

07. PUSHUPS MUFFINS

Prep: 15 Minutes
Cook Time: 30 Minutes
Total: 45 Minutes
Serves: 6

Ingredients

1 teaspoon coconut oil, for greasing muffin tins (optional)
2 tablespoons almond butter, or sunflower seed butter
¼ cup non-dairy milk
1 orange, peeled
1 carrot, coarsely chopped
2 tablespoons chopped dried apricots, or other dried fruit
3 tablespoons molasses

1 teaspoon pure vanilla extract
½ teaspoon ground cinnamon
½ teaspoon ground ginger (optional)
¼ teaspoon ground nutmeg (optional)
¼ teaspoon allspice (optional)
¾ cup rolled oats, or whole-grain flour
1 teaspoon baking powder
½ teaspoon baking soda
2 tablespoons ground flaxseed
1 teaspoon apple cider vinegar

Optional Mix-ins

½ cup rolled oats
2 tablespoons raisins, or other chopped dried fruit
2 tablespoons sunflower seeds

Preparation

Preparing the Ingredients.

Preheat the oven to 350°F.

Prepare a 6-cup muffin tin by rubbing the insides of the cups with coconut oil or using silicone or paper muffin cups.

Purée the nut butter, milk, orange, carrot, apricots, molasses, flaxseed, vinegar, vanilla, cinnamon, ginger, nutmeg, and allspice in a food processor or blender until somewhat smooth.

Grind the oats in a clean coffee grinder until they're the consistency of flour (or use whole-grain flour). In a large bowl, mix the oats with the baking powder and baking soda. Mix the wet ingredients into the dry ingredients until just combined. Fold in the mix-ins (if using). Spoon about ¼ cup batter into each muffin cup and bake for 30 minutes, or until a toothpick inserted into the center comes out clean.

The orange creates a very moist base, so the muffins may take longer than 30 minutes, depending on how heavy your muffin tin is. Store the muffins in the fridge or freezer, because they are so moist. If you plan to keep them frozen, you can easily double the batch for a full dozen.

Per Serving: Calories: 287; Protein: 8g; Total fat: 12g; Carbohydrates: 41g; Fiber: 6g

08. Vegan Tortilla Breakfast

Prep: 20 Minutes
Cook Time: 20 Minutes
Total: 40 Minutes
Serves: 6

Ingredients

Nonstick cooking spray
1 recipe Tofu-Spinach Scramble
1 (14-ounce) can black beans, rinsed and drained
¼ cup nutritional yeast

2 teaspoons hot sauce
10 small corn tortillas
½ cup shredded vegan Cheddar or pepper Jack cheese, divided

Preparation

Preparing the Ingredients.

Preheat the oven to 350°F.

Coat a 9-by-9-inch baking pan with cooking spray.

In a large bowl, combine the tofu scramble with the black beans, nutritional yeast, and hot sauce. Set aside.

In the bottom of the baking pan, place 5 corn tortillas. Spread half of the tofu and bean mixture over the tortillas. Spread ¼ cup of cheese over the top. Layer the remaining 5 tortillas over the top of the cheese. Spread the reminder of the tofu and bean mixture over the tortillas. Spread the remaining ¼ cup of cheese over the top.

Bake for 20 minutes. Divide evenly among 6 single-serving containers. Let cool before sealing the lids. Place the containers in the refrigerator for up to 5 days.

If you want to keep the casserole intact in the freezer, consider baking it in a disposable pan. Once cool, simply cover with foil and freeze.

Per Serving: Calories: 323; Protein: 27g; Carbohydrates: 60g; Fiber: 10g

09. Leg Day Pancakes

Prep: 10 Minutes
Cook Time: 15 Minutes
Total: 25 Minutes
Serves: 4

Ingredients

1 cup whole-wheat flour

1 teaspoon garlic salt

1 teaspoon onion powder

½ teaspoon baking soda

¼ teaspoon salt

1 cup lightly pressed, crumbled soft or firm tofu

⅓ cup unsweetened plant-based milk

¼ cup lemon juice (about 2 small lemons)

2 tablespoons extra-virgin olive oil

½ cup finely chopped mushrooms

½ cup finely chopped onion

2 cups tightly packed greens (arugula, spinach, or baby kale work great)

Nonstick cooking spray

Preparation

Preparing the Ingredients.

In a large bowl, combine the flour, garlic salt, onion powder, baking soda, and salt. Mix well. In a blender, combine the tofu, plant-based milk, lemon juice, and olive oil. Purée on high speed for 30 seconds.

Pour the contents of the blender into the bowl of dry ingredients and whisk until combined well. Fold in the mushrooms, onion, and greens.

Spray a large skillet or griddle pan with nonstick cooking spray and set over medium-high heat. Reduce the heat to medium and add ½ cup of batter per pancake. Cook on both sides for about 3 minutes, or until set. After flipping, press down on the cooked side of the pancake with a spatula to flatten out the pancake. Repeat until the batter is gone.

Divide the cooked pancakes among 4 single-serving containers. Let cool before sealing the lids.

Place the airtight storage containers in the refrigerator for up to 4 days. To reheat, microwave for 1½ to 2 minutes. To freeze, place the pancakes on a parchment paper–lined baking sheet in a single layer. If there's more than one layer, place another piece of parchment paper over the pancakes and place the second layer on top. Place the baking sheet in the freezer for 2 to 4 hours.

Transfer the frozen pancakes to a freezer-safe bag (cut the parchment paper and place a small piece between each pancake). To thaw, refrigerate overnight. Preheat an oven or toaster oven to 350°F. Place the pancakes on a parchment paper–lined baking sheet and bake for 10 to 15 minutes, or stack the pancakes on a plate and microwave for 2 to 3 minutes.

Per Serving: Calories: 246; Protein: 10g; Total fat: 11g; Carbohydrates: 30g; Fiber: 3g

10. Tropi-kale Morning Hero

Prep: 5 min
Cook Time: 0 min
Total: 5 min
Serves: 4

Ingredients

1 cup chopped pineapple (frozen or fresh)
1 cup chopped mango (frozen or fresh)
½ to 1 cup chopped kale
½ avocado

½ cup coconut milk
1 cup of water, or coconut water
1 teaspoon matcha green tea powder (optional)

Preparation

Preparing the Ingredients.

Pour everything in a blender until smooth, adding more water (or coconut milk) if needed.

Per Serving: Calories: 566; Protein: 8g; Total fat: 36g; Saturated fat: 1g; Carbohydrates: 66g; Fiber: 12g

11. BLUEBERRY OATMEAL BARS

Prep: 10 min
Cook time: 40 min
Total: 50 min
Serves: 12

Ingredients

2 cups uncooked rolled oats
2 cups all-purpose flour
1½ cups dark-brown sugar
1½ teaspoons baking soda
½ teaspoon sea salt

½ teaspoon ground cinnamon
1 cup vegan butter, melted
4 cups blueberries, fresh or frozen
¼ cup organic cane sugar
2 tablespoons cornstarch

Preparation

Preparing the Ingredients.

Preheat the oven to 375°F. Lightly grease a 9-by-13-inch baking dish.

In a large bowl, combine the oats, flour, sugar, baking soda, salt, and cinnamon. Add the butter and mix until well incorporated and crumbly.

In a separate large bowl, combine the blueberries, cane sugar, and cornstarch, mixing until the blueberries are evenly coated.

Press 3 cups of the oatmeal mixture into the prepared baking pan. Spread the blueberry mixture on top and crumble the remaining oatmeal mixture over the blueberries.

Bake for 40 minutes.

Remove from the oven and let cool completely before cutting into bars.

Per Serving: Calories: 160; Protein: 4g; Total fat: 2.5g; Saturated fat: 1g; Carbohydrates: 30g; Fiber: 6g

12. Quinoa Kettlebell Muffins

Prep: 10 Minutes
Cook Time: 15 Minutes
Total: 25 Minutes
Serves: 5

Ingredients

2 tablespoons coconut oil or margarine, melted, plus more for coating the muffin tin
¼ cup ground flaxseed
½ cup water
2 cups unsweetened applesauce
½ cup brown sugar

1 teaspoon apple cider vinegar
2½ cups whole-grain flour
1½ cups cooked quinoa
2 teaspoons baking soda
Pinch salt
½ cup dried cranberries or raisins

Preparation

Preheat the oven to 400°F.

Coat a muffin tin with coconut oil, line with paper muffin cups, or use a nonstick tin. In a large bowl, stir together the flaxseed and water. Add the applesauce, sugar, coconut oil, and vinegar. Stir to combine. Add the flour, quinoa, baking soda, and salt, stirring until just combined. Gently fold in the cranberries without stirring too much. Scoop the muffin mixture into the prepared tin, about ⅓ cup for each muffin.

Bake for 15 to 20 minutes, until lightly browned on top and springy to the touch. Let cool for about 10 minutes. Run a dinner knife around the inside of each cup to loosen, then tilt the muffins on their sides in the muffin wells so air gets underneath. These keep in an airtight container in the refrigerator for up to 1 week or in the freezer indefinitely.

Per Serving (1 muffin): Calories: 387; Protein: 7g; Total fat: 5g; Saturated fat: 2g; Carbohydrates: 57g; Fiber: 8g

13. Pumpkin Iron Pancakes

Prep: 15 Minutes
Cook Time: 15 Minutes
Total:30 Minutes
Serves: 4

Ingredients

2 cups unsweetened almond milk
1 teaspoon apple cider vinegar
2½ cups whole-wheat flour
2 tablespoons baking powder
½ teaspoon baking soda
1 teaspoon sea salt

1 teaspoon pumpkin pie spice or ½ teaspoon ground cinnamon plus
¼ teaspoon grated nutmeg plus ¼ teaspoon ground allspice
½ cup canned pumpkin purée
1 cup water
1 tablespoon coconut oil

Preparation

In a small bowl, combine the almond milk and apple cider vinegar. Set aside.

In a bowl, whisk together the flour, baking powder, baking soda, salt, and pumpkin pie spice. In the bowl, combine the almond milk mixture, pumpkin purée, and water, whisking to mix well. Mix the wet ingredients to the dry ingredients and fold together until the dry ingredients are just moistened.

In a nonstick pan or griddle over medium-high heat, melt the coconut oil and swirl to coat. Pour the batter into the pan ¼ cup at a time and cook until the pancakes are browned, about 5 minutes per side. Serve immediately.

Per Serving: Calories: 163; Protein: 8.5g; Total fat: 13.9g; Saturated fat: 2.4g; Carbohydrates: 4g; Fiber: 1.8g

14. QUINOA HERCULES BOWL

Prep: 5 Minutes
Cook Time: 0 Minutes
Total: 5 Minutes
Serves: 4

Ingredients

3 cups freshly cooked quinoa
1⅓ cups unsweetened soy or almond milk
2 bananas, sliced
1 cup raspberries

1 cup blueberries
½ cup chopped raw walnuts
¼ cup maple syrup

Preparation

Preparing the Ingredients

Divide the ingredients among 4 bowls, starting with a base of ¾ cup quinoa, ⅓ cup milk, ½ banana, ¼ cup raspberries, ¼ cup blueberries, and 2 tablespoons walnuts.

Drizzle 1 tablespoon of maple syrup over the top of each bowl.

Per Serving: Calories: 200; Protein: 24g; Total fat: 10.3g; Saturated fat: 1.2g; Carbohydrates: 109g; Fiber: 11.9g

15. Pull Up Pudding

Prep: 5 Minutes
Cook Time: 50 Minutes
Total: 55 Minutes
Serves: 4

Ingredients

1 cup rice
1½ cups water
1½ cups non dairy milk
3 tablespoons sugar (omit if using a
sweetened non dairy milk)

2 teaspoons pumpkin pie spice or
ground cinnamon
2 bananas
3 tablespoons chopped walnuts or
sunflower seeds (optional)

Preparation

Preparing the Ingredients.

In a medium pot, combine the rice, water, milk, sugar, and pumpkin pie spice. Bring to a boil over high heat, turn the heat to low, and cover the pot. Simmer, stirring occasionally, until the rice is soft and the liquid is absorbed. White rice takes about 20 minutes; brown rice takes about 50 minutes.

Smash the bananas and stir them into the cooked rice. Serve topped with walnuts (if using). Leftovers will keep refrigerated in an airtight container for up to 5 days.

Per Serving: Calories: 479; Protein: 9g; Total fat: 13g; Saturated fat: 1g; Carbohydrates: 86g; Fiber: 7g

16. Ten More Reps Parfaits

Prep: 15 min
Cook Time: 0 min
Total: 15 min
Serves: 2

Ingredients

One 14-ounce can coconut milk, refrigerated overnight
1 cup granola

½ cup walnuts
1 cup sliced strawberries or other seasonal berries

Preparation

Pour off the canned coconut-milk liquid and retain the solids.

In two parfait glasses, layer the coconut-milk solids, granola, walnuts, and strawberries. Serve immediately.

Per Serving : Calories: 332; Protein: 3.14g; Total fat: 15.44g; Carbohydrates: 40g; Fiber: 0.9g

17. Orange Couscous Boss Breakfast

Prep: 10 min
Cook Time: 10 min
Total: 20 min
Serves: 4

Ingredients

3 cups orange juice
1 ½ cups couscous
1 teaspoon ground cinnamon
1 cup adzuki beans boiled

¼ teaspoon ground cloves
½ cup dried fruit, such as raisins or apricots
½ cup chopped almonds or other nuts or seeds

Preparation

Preparing the Ingredients.

In a small saucepan, bring the orange juice to a boil. Add the couscous, cinnamon, and cloves and remove from heat. Cover the pan with a lid and allow to sit until the couscous softens, about 5 minutes.

Fluff the couscous with a fork and stir in the adzuki beans, dried fruit and nuts. Serve immediately.

Per Serving: Calories: 130; Protein: 9g; Total fat: 9g; Carbohydrates: 10g; Fiber: 3g

18. THE HULK TACO SALAD

Prep: 10 min
Cook Time: 2 min
Total: 12 min
Serves: 4

Ingredients

4 tablespoons tahini
1 teaspoon maple syrup or agave nectar
4 tablespoons olive oil
2 cups cooked or canned black beans
1 avocado, peeled, pitted, diced

4 teaspoons chili powder
Juice of 2 limes
2 cups chopped cherry tomatoes
1 cup cooked corn, fresh or frozen
8 cups Romaine lettuce or any other greens of your choice

Preparation

Add all the ingredients for dressing into a small jar. Fasten the lid and shake the jar vigorously until well combined. Add water to dilute if desired. Refrigerate until use.

Add all the ingredients for salad into a bowl and toss well. Drizzle the dressing on top. Toss well and serve.

Per Serving: Calories: 703; Protein: 28g; Total fat: 31g; Carbohydrates: 87g; Fiber: 25g

19. Tempeh Miracules Muffin

Prep: 5 min
Cook Time: 7 min
Total: 12 min
Serves: 1

Ingredients

1 ½ tablespoons soy sauce or tamari
½ tablespoon apple cider vinegar
½ teaspoon smoked paprika
¾ tablespoon maple syrup
2 small cloves garlic, minced
Pepper to taste
1 vegan English muffin, split, toasted

¼ avocado, peeled, pitted, sliced
Dijon mustard to taste
Ketchup
A handful baby spinach
½ tablespoon olive oil
4 ounces tempeh, cut into 2 – 3 thin slices

Preparation

Add all the ingredients for sauce into a small bowl and stir.

Place a skillet over medium heat. Add oil.

When the oil is heated, place tempeh in a single layer and cook until the underside is brown. Flip sides and cook the other side until brown.

Add the sauce mixture and stir until well coated. Cook until dry. Flip the tempeh a couple of times while cooking.

Spread a little ketchup and Dijon mustard over the cut part of the English muffin.

Place tempeh slices on the bottom half of the muffins. Place avocado slices and baby spinach.

Cover with the top half of the English muffin and serve.

Per Serving: Calories: 573; Protein: 29.1g; Total fat: 30.3g; Carbohydrates: 54g; Fiber: 6.4g

20. Fig And Tofu Oatmeal

Prep: 10 min
Cook Time: 0 min
Total: 10 min
Serves: 1

Ingredients

½ cup water
½ cup rolled oats
Pinch salt
2 tablespoons dried figs, sliced

2 tablespoons soft tofu
2 teaspoons maple syrup
1 tablespoon almonds, toasted and sliced

Preparation

Put the water, oats and salt in a glass jar with a lid.

Shake to blend well.

Refrigerate for up to 5 days.

Top with the remaining ingredients when ready to serve. Nutritional Value:

Per Serving: Calories: 294; Protein: 10.4g; Total fat: 2.3g; Carbohydrates: 47.5g; Fiber: 6.6g

21. LOAD-IT-UP! FAJITAS

Prep: 10 min
Cook Time: 12 min
Total: 22 min
Serves: 2

Ingredients

2 large Portobello mushrooms, cut into thick slices
1 ½ red bell peppers, thinly sliced
½ pound extra-firm tofu, chopped
1 onion, thinly sliced

1 tablespoon lime juice
½ tablespoon coconut oil
½ tablespoon taco seasoning
¼ cup chopped cilantro

Preparation

Place a skillet over medium heat. Add oil. When the oil is heated, add onion and bell pepper and sauté until slightly tender.

Add tofu and cook for a couple of minutes. Stir in the mushrooms and taco seasoning. Cook until vegetables are soft.

Add lime juice and salt and mix well. Remove from heat.

Serve over tortillas with toppings of your choice.

Per serving: Without tortillas or toppings Calories:335, Fat:15g, Total Carbohydrate :31 g, Protein :18.5 g

22. ONE-UP TOFU

Prep: 5 min
Cook Time: 40 min
Total: 45 min (2-3 hours additional)
Serves: 4

Ingredients

Extra firm tofu – 28 ounces
Vegan barbeque sauce – as per taste
Vegan teriyaki sauce – as per taste
Tofu cutlets
Soy sauce (low sodium) - 2 tablespoons
Garlic powder (divided) - ¾ teaspoon
All-purpose flour - ½ cup
Corn starch - 1 tablespoon

Non-dairy milk (unsweetened) - ½ cup
Panko bread crumbs - ½ cup
Nutritional yeast - 1 tablespoon
Paprika - 1 teaspoon
Cayenne pepper - ¼ teaspoon
Kosher salt - ½ teaspoon
Pepper - ¼ teaspoon
Olive oil – as required

Preparation

Start by preheating the oven by setting the temperature to 400 degrees Fahrenheit.

Take 2 tofu blocks and slice them through the center. Place all the blocks on the kitchen towel and cover with another. Place a baking tray and a heavy object to drain excess liquid. Let it sit for about an hour.

Take 2 tofu blocks and place them on a baking dish. Drizzle low-sodium soy sauce over each side evenly. Sprinkle gently with ¼ teaspoon of garlic powder on each side. Coat evenly. Let the tofu marinate for about 10 minutes.

Take a small mixing bowl and add in the cornstarch and flour. Mix well to combine. Take another bowl and pour in the milk.

Take a third mixing bowl and toss in the nutritional yeast, bread crumbs, paprika, cayenne pepper, remaining garlic powder, pepper and salt. Mix well to combine.

Take the marinated tofu and coat it with cornstarch mixture and then dip it in milk. Again coat it in cornstarch mixture, dip in milk and finish by coating it with bread crumb and spice mixture.

Repeat the procedure with the second tofu block.

Take a baking dish and lightly grease it with olive oil. Place the tofu blocks and brush them using olive oil on each side.

Take the non-breaded tofu pieces and place them on the baking dish.

Take the teriyaki sauce and brush it on both sides of one non-breaded tofu piece.

Take the barbeque sauce and brush it on both sides of one non-breaded tofu piece.

Place the baking dish in the preheated oven and cook for about 15 minutes. Flip all the four pieces and cook for another 15 minutes.

Remove the baking dish from the oven and transfer the tofu cutlets onto a wooden chopping board. Cut into cubes.

Serve them with salads or use them in sandwiches or wraps.

Note – These baked tofu cutlets can be stored in the refrigerator for up to 5 days.

Per serving; calories: 350 Fat:17 g, Carbohydrates:28 g, Protein:24 g,

23. PORRIDGE WITH BLUEBERRY COMPOTE

Preparation time: 5 min
Cook time: 5 min
Total time: 10 min
Serves: 2

Ingredients

6 tbsp porridge oats
½ cup soy yogurt

1/2 * 350 g pack frozen blueberries
1 tsp maple syrup

Preparations

In a non-stick pan put 400mL water along with oats. Cook over the heat. Stir it occasionally for about 2 minutes until it comes in thickened consistency. Remove from the heat.

Add a third of the yogurt.

Tip the blueberries into a pan with 1 tbsp water and maple syrup. Poach them gently until the blueberries have thawed and get tender. Make sure they stay tender but still hold their shape.

Pour the porridge into bowls. Top with the remaining yogurt and spoon over the blueberries.

Per Serving : Calories: 214; Protein: 13g; Total fat: 4g; Carbohydrates: 35g; Fiber: 7g

24. VEGAN APPLE PANCAKES

Preparation time: 10 min
Cook time: 10 min
Total time: 20 min
Serves: 4 to 5 servings

Ingredients

1 cups soy milk-1/2 cups,(or other vegan milk)
½ cup tofu, Soft/Silken
1/3 cup vegetable shortening
½ cup flour
2--½ tsp baking powder
½ tsp salt

½ tsp cinnamon
½ tsp nutmeg
2 apples, chopped
1/3 cup pecans, chopped
2 tbsp oil, more or less as needed for frying

Preparation

Gather all the ingredients. In a blender or food processor, add all ingredients except pecans until apples are minced. Blend all the ingredients.

Gently fold in the pecans.

Drop by a large spoonful onto a lightly oiled skillet or griddle. Cook for a few minutes until bubbles appear. Flip and cook until both sides are lightly golden brown.

Your dish is ready to serve.

Per Serving: Calories: 381; Protein: 8g; Total fat: 25g; Carbohydrates: 34g; Fiber: 5g

25. MEXICAN BEANS & AVOCADO ON TOAST

Preparation time: 20 min
Cook time: 10 min
Total time: 30 min
Serves: 4 servings

Ingredients

Quartered cherry potatoes, 270g
1 red or white onion finely chopped
½ lime juice
4 tbsp olive oil
2 garlic cloves, crushed
1 tsp ground cumin
2 tsp chipotle paste or 1 tsp chilli flakes

*2*400g cans black beans, drained*
Small bunch coriander, chopped
4 slices bread
1 avocado, finely sliced

Preparations

In a bowl mix the tomatoes, ¼ onion, lime juice and 1 tbsp oil and set aside. Fry the remaining onion in 2 tbsp oil until it starts to soften. Now add the garlic and fry for 1 minute, add cumin, chipotle and stir until it gets fragrant.

Tip in the beans and a splash of water, stir and cook gently until heated through.

Now stir in the tomato mixture and cook for 1 minute. Season well and add most of the coriander.

Now toast the bread, drizzle it with the remaining 1 tbsp oil. Put a slice on each plate and pile some beans on top. Arrange some spices of avocado on top.

Sprinkle with the remaining tomato mixture and coriander leaves to serve.

Per Serving: Calories: 368; Protein: 12g; Total fat: 19g; Carbohydrates: 30g; Fiber: 13g

26. No Yeast Cinnamon Rolls

Preparation time: 15 min
Cook time: 25 min
Total time: 40 min
Serves: 8 rolls or 8 servings

Ingredients

For the Dough:

4 tablespoons melted unsalted butter, divided
2 1/2 cups all-purpose flour
2 tablespoons granulated sugar
1 1/4 teaspoons baking powder
1/2 teaspoon baking soda
1/2 teaspoon salt
1 cup nut butter
1/4 cup almond milk

For the Filling:

1/4 cup nut butter, softened
1 cup firmly packed brown sugar
1 tablespoon ground cinnamon

For the Icing:

1 cup powdered sugar
3 tablespoons nut butter, softened
3 ounces vegan cream cheese, softened
1 tablespoon almond milk
1/2 teaspoon vanilla extract

Preparation

Preheat the oven at 425 F temperature. Grease the bottom of a 9 inch round cake pan with melted nut butter. Leave it aside.

In a large bowl whisk together flour, sugar, baking powder, baking soda and salt. Now add nut butter, almond milk and 2 more tbsp of the melted nut butter to the flour mixture.

45

Stir until it all combines together with each other. Start kneading it with your hands for 30 seconds. The dough will be sticky.

Prepare a lightly floured work surface, now roll out the dough into a 12*10 inch rectangle.

Spread ¼ cup of the softened nut butter onto the entire surface of the dough. Spread brown sugar and cinnamon evenly onto dough.

Press the filling into the dough very lightly. Roll the dough to form a log shape starting with the long end of the rectangle to the opposite end. Now cut the dough into 8 equal sections.

Place one roll in the center of the prepared cake pan followed by placing the remaining seven rolls evenly around the first.

Brush the tops with remaining 1 tbsp of melted nut butter.

Place rolls in the preheated oven and bake for 15 minutes then reduce the temperature to 350F—allow it to bake it for 10 minutes more until it is lightly browned.

Meanwhile, prepare the icing.

In a large bowl of a stand mixer, combine the powdered sugar, softened nut butter, softened vegan cream cheese, almond milk and vanilla extract until light and creamy.

Remove the cinnamon rolls from the oven and allow it to cool for 5 to 10 minutes before spreading the cream cheese icing on top.

Serve immediately.

Note: the cinnamon rolls can be stored in an airtight container for 2 days.

Per Serving: Calories: 401.7; Protein: 5g; Total fat: 18g; Carbohydrates: 54g; Fiber: 1.4g

LUNCHES

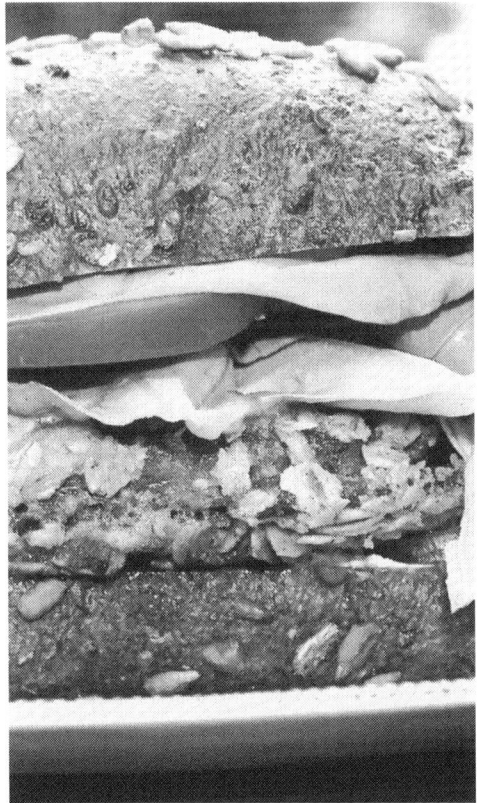

You should keep your metabolism active all day.

This is especially true if you work out more than once in a day. You can surely have snacks during the day, but lunch is a fundamental moment to fuel up in the middle of your day.

27. GEAR UP LENTILS

Prep: 5 min
Cook Time: 40 min
Total: 45 min
Serves: 6

Ingredients

5 cups water
2¼ cups dry French or brown lentils, rinsed
and drained
3 teaspoons minced garlic (about 3 cloves)
1 bay leaf

½ teaspoon dried basil
½ teaspoon dried oregano
½ teaspoon dried rosemary
½ teaspoon dried thyme

Preparation

In a large pot, combine the water, lentils, garlic, bay leaf, basil, oregano, rosemary, and thyme. Bring to a boil. Reduce the heat to low, cover, and simmer for 25 to 40 minutes, until tender, stirring occasionally. Drain any excess cooking liquid.

Transfer to a container, or scoop 1 cup of lentils into each of 6 storage containers. Let cool before sealing the lids.

Place the containers in the refrigerator for up to 5 days.

Per Serving (1 cup): Calories: 257; Fat: 1g; Protein: 19g; Carbohydrates: 44g; Fiber: 22g; Sugar: 2g; Sodium: 5mg

28. CAULIFLOWER TACOS

Prep: 10 min
Cook Time: 30 min
Total: 40 min
Serves: 8

Ingredients

For The Roasted Cauliflower

1 head cauliflower, cut into bite-size pieces
1 tablespoon olive oil (optional)
2 tablespoons whole-grain flour
1 to 2 teaspoons smoked paprika

2 tablespoons nutritional yeast
½ to 1 teaspoon chili powder
Pinch sea salt

For The Tacos

2 cups shredded lettuce
2 cups cherry tomatoes, quartered
2 carrots, scrubbed or peeled, and grated
½ cup Fresh Mango Salsa

½ cup Guacamole
8 small whole-grain or corn tortillas
1 lime, cut into 8 wedges

Preparation

To make the roasted cauliflower

Preheat the oven to 350°F. Lightly grease a large rectangular baking sheet with olive oil, or line it with parchment paper. In a large bowl, toss the cauliflower pieces with oil (if using), or just rinse them so they're wet. The idea is to get the seasonings to stick. In a smaller bowl, mix together the flour, nutritional yeast, paprika, chili powder, and salt.

Add the seasonings to the cauliflower, and mix it around with your hands to thoroughly coat. Spread the cauliflower on the baking sheet, and roast for 20 to 30 minutes, or until softened.

To make the tacos:

Prep the veggies, salsa, and guacamole while the cauliflower is roasting. Once the cauliflower is cooked, heat the tortillas for just a few minutes in the oven or in a small skillet. Set everything out on the table, and assemble your tacos as you go. Give a squeeze of fresh lime just before eating.

Per Serving (1 taco): Calories: 198; Total fat: 6g; Carbs: 32g; Fiber: 6g; Protein: 7g

29. BOULDERS BEAN BURGERS

Prep: 10 min
Cook Time: 10 min
Total: 20 min
Serves: 4

Ingredients

*1 tablespoon olive oil, plus more for coating
the baking sheet*
¼ cup couscous
¼ cup boiling water
*1 (15-ounce) can white beans, drained and
rinsed*
2 tablespoons balsamic vinegar
*2 tablespoons chopped sun-dried tomatoes or
olives*

*½ teaspoon garlic powder or 1 garlic
clove, finely minced*
½ teaspoon salt
4 burger buns
Lettuce leaves, for serving
Tomato slices, for serving
*Condiments of choice, such as ketchup,
olive tapenade, Creamy Tahini
Dressing , and/or Spinach Pesto*

Preparation

If baking, preheat the oven to 350°F.

Coat a rimmed baking sheet with olive oil or line it with parchment paper or a
silicone mat. In a medium heat-proof bowl, combine the couscous and boiling water.

Cover and set aside for about 5 minutes. Once the couscous is soft and the water
is absorbed, fluff it with a fork. Add the beans, and mash them to a chunky texture.
Add the vinegar, olive oil, sun-dried tomatoes, garlic powder, and salt; stir until
combined but still a bit chunky.

Divide the mixture into 4 portions, and shape each into a patty. Put the patties
on the prepared baking sheet, and bake for 25 to 30 minutes, until slightly crispy on

the edges. Alternatively, heat some olive oil in a large skillet over medium heat, then add the patties, making sure each has oil under it.

Fry for about 5 minutes, until the bottoms are browned. Flip, adding more oil as needed, and fry for about 5 minutes more. Serve the burgers on buns with lettuce, tomato, and your choice of condiments.

Per Serving: Calories: 314; Total fat: 4g; Carbs: 53.79g; Fiber: 11.8g; Protein: 15.88g

30. BLACK BEAN PIZZA PLATE

Prep: 10 min
Cook Time: 20 min
Total: 30 min
Serves: 2

Ingredients

2 prebaked pizza crusts
½ cup Spicy Black Bean Dip
1 tomato, thinly sliced
Pinch freshly ground black pepper

1 carrot, grated
Pinch sea salt
1 red onion, thinly sliced
1 avocado, sliced

Preparation

Preheat the oven to 400°F.

Lay the two crusts out on a large baking sheet. Spread half the Spicy Black Bean Dip on each pizza crust.

Then layer on the tomato slices with a pinch pepper if you like. Sprinkle the grated carrot with the sea salt and lightly massage it in with your hands.

Spread the carrot on top of the tomato, then add the onion.

Pop the pizzas in the oven for 10 to 20 minutes, or until they're done to your taste. Top the cooked pizzas with sliced avocado and another sprinkle of pepper.

Per Serving (1 pizza): Calories: 379; Total fat: 13g; Carbs: 59g; Fiber: 15g; Protein: 13g

31. Hulk'n'bulk Wrap

Prep: 15 min
Cook Time: 0 min
Total: 15 min
Serves: 3

Ingredients

3 tablespoons tahini
Zest and juice of 1 lime
1 tablespoon curry powder
¼ teaspoon sea salt
3 to 4 tablespoons water
1 (14-ounce) can chickpeas, rinsed and drained, or 1½ cups cooked

1 cup diced mango
1 red bell pepper, seeded and diced small
½ cup fresh cilantro, chopped3 large whole-grain wraps
1 to 2 cups shredded green leaf lettuce

Preparation

In a medium bowl, whisk together the tahini, lime zest and juice, curry powder, and salt until the mixture is creamy and thick.

Add 3 to 4 tablespoons of water to thin it out a bit. Or you can process this all in a blender. The taste should be strong and salty, to flavor the whole salad.

Toss the chickpeas, mango, bell pepper, and cilantro with the tahini dressing. Spoon the salad down the center of the wraps, top with shredded lettuce, and then roll up and enjoy.

Per Serving (1 wrap): Calories: 437; Total fat: 8g; Carbs: 79g; Fiber: 12g; Protein: 15g

32. Rice Broccoli Bake

Prep: 10 min
Cook Time: 40 min
Total: 50 min
Serves: 7

Ingredients

2 cups cooked brown rice
1 (12-ounce) bag frozen broccoli florets, chopped, or 2 cups chopped fresh broccoli florets

½ cup chopped onion
1 celery stalk, thinly sliced
1 batch Vegan Cheese Sauce

Preparation

Preparing the Ingredients.

Preheat the oven to 425°F.

In a large bowl, mix together the rice, broccoli, onion, celery, and vegan cheese sauce. Transfer to a 2-quart or 8-inch-square baking dish.

Bake for 40 minutes, or until the top has started to brown slightly.

Serve.

Per Serving: Calories: 287; Total fat: 13.02g; Carbs: 32.01g; Fiber: 2.7g; Protein: 11.13g

33. GRAIN GREEN AND BEAN BOWL

Prep: 10 min
Cook Time: 5 min
Total: 15 min
Serves: 2

Ingredients

2 teaspoons olive oil
1 cup cooked brown rice, quinoa, or your grain of choice
1 (15-ounce) can chickpeas or your beans of choice, rinsed and drained

1 bunch spinach or kale, stemmed and roughly chopped
1 tablespoon soy sauce or gluten-free tamari
Sea salt
Black pepper

Preparation

In a large skillet, heat the oil over medium heat.

Add the rice, beans, and greens and stir continuously until the greens have wilted and everything is heated through, 3 to 5 minutes. Drizzle in the soy sauce, mix to combine, and season with salt and pepper.

Per Serving: Calories: 158; Total fat: 10g; Carbs: 28g; Fiber: 5g; Protein: 6.8g

34. RATATOUILLE

Prep: 25 min
Cook Time: 4 hrs
Total: 4 hrs 25 min
Serves: 6

Ingredients

1 cup dry lentils, rinsed and drained
1 small eggplant (12 ounces), peeled and cubed
2 (14.5 ounce) cans diced tomatoes with basil, garlic and oregano, undrained
2 large onions, coarsely chopped

2 medium yellow summer squash and/or zucchini, halved lengthwise and cut into ½-inch-thick slices (about 2 ½ cups)
1 medium red sweet pepper, seeded and chopped
½ cup water
¼ to ½ teaspoon ground black pepper

Preparation

Preparing the Ingredients. On your electric pressure cooker, select Sauté. Add the onion, garlic, and olive oil. Cook for 4 to 5 minutes, stirring occasionally, until the onion is softened.

Add the water, tomatoes, eggplant, zucchini, bell peppers, and herbes de Provence. Cancel Sauté.

High pressure for 6 minutes. Close and lock the lid, and select High Pressure for 6 minutes.

Pressure Release. Once the cook time is complete, let the pressure release naturally, about 20 minutes. Unlock and remove the lid. Let cool for a few minutes, then season with salt and pepper.

In a 3 1/2- or 4-quart slow cooker, combine lentils, eggplant, undrained tomatoes, onions, summer squash, sweet pepper, water and black pepper. Cover and cook on a low-heat setting for 8 to 9 hours or on a high-heat setting for 4 to 4 1/2 hours.

Per serving: Calories: 215; Total fat: 1g; Protein: 12g; Sodium: 42mg; Fiber: 12g

35. Lemon And Thyme Couscous

Prep: 15 min
Cook Time: 20 min
Total: 35 min
Serves: 1

Ingredients

1 Zucchini
4 oz Grape Tomatoes
1/4 oz Fresh Thyme
2 Green Onion
2 cloves Garlic
1 Lemon 1
7 oz Boiled Chickpeas
1 tsp Smoked Paprika

3/4 cup Pearl Couscous
1.5 cup Veggie Stock
1/2 cup fresh tofu
2 tsp Olive Oil
1 tbsp Butter
1.25 tsp Salt
Pepper

Preparation

Preheat the oven to 425 degrees Fahrenheit.

Wash all the vegetables and prepare them to be chopped. Cut zucchini into 1/2 inch cubes and halve the tomatoes. Strip thyme leaves from their stems. Thinly slice green onions, keeping green and white parts separate.

Mince garlic and halve lemon.

Toss tomatoes, zucchini and half of thyme on a baking sheet with a drizzle of olive oil. Season with 1/2 tsp of salt and 1/4 tsp of pepper. Roast in the middle rack for about 20 minutes, tossing half way through.

Drain and rinse chickpeas if it is canned. On another baking sheet combine chickpeas, 1 tbsp olive oil, paprika, salt, and pepper. Bake it in the oven for 20 minutes in the middle rack, tossing half way through until crisp.

In a saucepan heat butter, add white portion of the green onions and garlic minced. Once they are cooked, add couscous and the thyme leaves. Toss to coat, season it with salt and pepper according to need, continue stirring until couscous are lightly roasted.

Add about 1.5 cup of stock and let it boil. Now reduce the heat and cook until the liquid is absorbed, uncovered.

Now add half the veggies, half the fresh tofu, and squeeze a lemon to couscous pot, mix all gently.

Divide the couscous mixture in a plate. Top it with remaining chickpeas, veggies, and tofu. Sprinkle green part of onion. And your dish is ready to serve.

Per Serving: Calories: 460; Total fat: 9.9g; Carbs: 82g; Fiber: 14g; Protein: 17g

36. Quinoa Sushi

Prep: 2 min
Cook Time: 25 min
Total: 27 min
Serves: 4

Ingredients

2 cups water

1 cup dry quinoa, rinsed

¼ cup unseasoned rice vinegar

¼ cup mirin or white wine vinegar

Preparation

In a large saucepan, bring the water to a boil. Add the quinoa to the boiling water, stir, cover, and reduce the heat to low. Simmer for 15 to 20 minutes, until the liquid is absorbed. Remove from the heat and let stand for 5 minutes.

Fluff with a fork. Add the vinegar and mirin, and stir to combine well.

Divide the quinoa evenly among 4 mason jars or single-serving containers. Let cool before sealing the lids.

Per Serving: *Calories: 192; Fat: 3g; Protein: 6g; Carbohydrates: 34g; Fiber: 3g; Sugar: 4g; Sodium: 132mg*

37. LENTIL SPINACH CURRY

Prep: 5 min
Cook Time: 30 min
Total: 35 min
Serves: 4

Ingredients

1 teaspoon olive oil
1 onion, chopped
½-inch piece fresh ginger, peeled and minced
1 to 2 tablespoons mild curry powder
1½ cups dried green or brown lentils
2½ cups water or Economical Vegetable Broth

1 cup canned diced tomatoes
2 to 4 cups finely chopped raw spinach
½ cup non dairy milk
2 tablespoons soy sauce (optional)
1 tablespoon apple cider vinegar or rice vinegar
1 teaspoon salt (or 2 teaspoons if omitting soy sauce)

Preparation

Heat the olive oil in a pot over medium heat. Add the onion, and sauté for about 3 minutes, until soft.

Add the ginger, cook for 1 minute more. Stir in the curry powder, lentils, and water. Bring to a boil, turn the heat to low, and cover the pot. Simmer for 15 to 20 minutes, until the lentils are soft.

Stir in the tomatoes, spinach, milk, soy sauce (if using), vinegar, and salt. Simmer for about 3 minutes, until heated through. If you prefer, use an immersion blender to half-blend this in the pot for a creamier texture and to hide the spinach.

Store in a container for 4 to 5 days in the refrigerator or up to 1 month in the freezer.

Per Serving: Calories: 313; Protein: 21g; Total fat: 3g; Saturated fat: 0g; Carbohydrates: 52g; Fiber: 24g

38. GUN SHOW BARLEY STEW

Prep: 15 min
Cook Time: 20 min
Total: 45 min
Serves: 6

Ingredients

2 or 3 parsnips, peeled and chopped
2 cups chopped peeled sweet potato, russet potato, winter squash, or pumpkin
1 large yellow onion, chopped
1 cup pearl barley
1 (28-ounce) can diced tomatoes

4 cups water or unsalted vegetable broth
2 to 3 teaspoons dried mixed herbs or 1 teaspoon dried basil plus 1 teaspoon dried oregano
Salt
Freshly ground black pepper

Preparation

In your pot, combine the parsnips, sweet potato, onion, barley, tomatoes with their juice, water, and herbs.

High pressure for 20 minutes. Close and lock the lid, and select High Pressure for 20 minutes.

Pressure Release. Select quick release, being careful not to get your fingers or face near the steam release. Unlock and remove the lid. Taste and season with salt and pepper.

Per Serving: Calories: 300; Protein: 9g; Total fat: 2g; Carbohydrates: 16; Fiber: 14g

39. Power Mushroom Stroganoff

Prep: 10 min
Cook Time: 15 min
Total: 25 min
Serves: 6

Ingredients

1 tablespoon olive oil
1 onion, chopped
2 (8-ounce) packages baby bella or white button mushrooms, stemmed and sliced
4 garlic cloves, minced
¼ cup low-sodium vegetable broth
1 teaspoon paprika

½ teaspoon sea salt
½ teaspoon black pepper
¼ cup Sour Cream or store-bought vegan sour cream
4 tablespoons chopped fresh parsley, divided
1 pound lentil pasta of your choice, cooked

Preparation

Preparing the Ingredients.

Heat the oil in a large skillet over medium heat.

Add the onion and mushrooms and sauté for 5 to 8 minutes, until the mushrooms are soft and have reduced in size.

Add the garlic and sauté for 1 additional minute, or until fragrant.

Add the broth, paprika, salt, and pepper and cook for 5 more minutes, or until well incorporated and heated through.

Remove from the heat and stir in the sour cream and 2 tablespoons of parsley.

Toss with the cooked pasta, divide into 6 portions, and sprinkle with the remaining 2 tablespoons of parsley.

Per Serving: Calories: 400; Protein: 10g; Total fat: 12g; Carbohydrates: 61; Fiber: 6g

40. Maxing Out Balsamic Black Beans

Prep: 5 min
Cook Time: 20 min
Total: 25 min
Serves: 5

Ingredients

1 teaspoon extra-virgin olive oil or vegetable broth
½ cup diced sweet onion
1 teaspoon ground cumin
1 teaspoon ground cardamom (optional)

2 (14.5-ounce) cans black beans, rinsed and drained
¼ to ½ cup vegetable broth
2 tablespoons balsamic vinegar

Preparation

In a large pot over medium-high heat, heat the olive oil.

Add the onion, cumin, and cardamom (if using) and sauté for 3 to 5 minutes, until the onion is translucent.

Add the beans and ¼ cup broth, and bring to a boil. Add up to ½ cup more of broth for "soupier" beans.

Cover, reduce the heat, and simmer for 10 minutes. Add the balsamic vinegar, increase the heat to medium-high, and cook for 3 more minutes uncovered.

Transfer to a large storage container, or divide the beans evenly among 5 single-serving storage containers. Let cool before sealing the lids.

Place the containers in the refrigerator for up to 5 days .

Per Serving: Calories: 200; Fat: 2g; Protein: 13g; Carbohydrates: 34g; Fiber: 12g; Sugar: 1g; Sodium: 41mg

41. Rice and Lentils Overload

Prep: 10 min
Cook Time: 15 min
Total: 25 min
Serves: 4

Ingredients

2 tablespoons olive oil
1 onion, diced
1 carrot, diced
1 celery stalk, diced
2 15-ounce cans lentils, drained and rinsed
1 15-ounce can diced tomatoes with juice

1 tablespoon dried rosemary
1 tablespoon garlic powder
2 cups prepared brown rice
Sea salt
Freshly ground black pepper

Preparation

In a large pot, heat the olive oil over medium-high heat until it shimmers.

Add the onion, carrot, and celery and cook until the vegetables soften, about 5 minutes.

Add the lentils, tomatoes, rosemary, and garlic powder. Lower the heat to medium-low and simmer to blend the flavors, 5 to 7 minutes.

Stir the rice into lentils and heat through, 2 to 3 minutes. Season with salt and pepper and serve immediately.

Per serving: Calories: 332; Protein: 13.5g; Carbs: 63g; Fat: 3.4g; Fiber: 8.9g

42. Chickpeas Gainz Burgers

Prep: 20 min
Cook Time: 30 min
Total: 50 min
Serves: 12

Ingredients

1 red bell pepper
1 (19-ounce) can chickpeas, rinsed and drained, or 2 cups cooked
1 cup ground almonds
2 teaspoons Dijon mustard
2 teaspoons maple syrup
1 garlic clove, pressed

Juice of ½ lemon
1 teaspoon dried oregano
½ teaspoon dried sage
1 cup spinach
1 to 1½ cups rolled oats

Preparation

Preheat the oven to 350°F.

Line a large baking sheet with parchment paper.

Cut the red pepper in half, remove the stem and seeds, and put on the baking sheet cut side up in the oven. Roast in the oven while you prep the other ingredients.

Put the chickpeas in the food processor, along with the almonds, mustard, maple syrup, garlic, lemon juice, oregano, sage, and spinach. Pulse until things thoroughly combined but not puréed.

When the red pepper is softened a bit, about 10 minutes, add it to the processor along with the oats and pulse until they are chopped just enough to form patties.

If you don't have a food processor, mash the chickpeas with a potato masher or fork, and make sure everything else is chopped up as finely as possible, then stir together.

Scoop up ¼-cup portions and form into 12 patties, and lay them out on the baking sheet. Put the burgers in the oven and bake until the outside is lightly browned, about 30 minutes.

Per Serving (1 burger): Calories: 200; Total fat: 11g; Carbs: 21g; Fiber: 6g; Protein: 8g

43. HIRT CURRY QUINOA

Prep: 10 min
Cook Time: 20 min
Total: 30 min
Serves: 3

Ingredients

½ *tablespoon olive oil*
1 *small green bell pepper, deseeded, chopped*
1 *medium yellow onion, chopped*
1 *small sweet potato, chopped (about ¾ cup)*
½ *tablespoon red curry paste*
½ *cup quinoa*

1 *tablespoon lime juice*
A handful fresh cilantro, chopped
1 *clove garlic, chopped*
1 *teaspoon fresh ginger, peeled, chopped*
2 *cups vegetable broth or water*
Salt to taste

Preparation

Place a pot over medium-high heat. Add oil. When the oil is heated, add onion, sweet potato and bell pepper. Sauté for about 10 minutes.

Stir in ginger, garlic and curry paste. Sauté until aromatic.

Add quinoa and stir-fry for a minute.

Add broth and stir.

When it begins to boil, lower the heat and cook until sweet potatoes and quinoa are cooked.

Turn off the heat. Stir in lime juice and salt.

Ladle into soup bowls. Sprinkle cilantro on top and serve.

Per serving: Calories:164; Fat: 4g; Carbohydrate: 26g; Fiber: NA; Protein: 6 g

44. Split Pea Soup

Prep: 10 min
Cook Time: 10 min
Total: 20 min
Serves: 3

Ingredients

½ tablespoon canola oil
1 medium white onion, finely chopped
1 small stalk celery, sliced
2 cups vegetable broth
¾ cups green split peas, rinsed
½ small russet potato, cubed

½ teaspoon ground cumin
Freshly ground pepper to taste
1 cup water
Salt to taste
1 small carrot, chopped

Preparation

Place a soup pot over medium heat. Add oil. When the oil is heated, add onion, garlic, celery, and carrots and sauté for 3-4 minutes.

Add the rest of the ingredients in a large pot and stir.

Cook until the split peas and potatoes are tender. Add more water if required.

Mix well. Ladle into soup bowls and serve hot.

Per serving: Calories:163; Fat: 3g; Carbohydrate: 29g; Fiber: 5g; Protein:7 g

45. Under The Bar Burritos

Prep: 3 min
Cook Time: 1 min
Total: 4 min
Serves: 2

Ingredients

1½ cups (390 g) Slow-Cooker Refried Beans
1 large sweet potato, cubed and roasted or steamed
½ cup (30 g) nutritional yeast

½ cup (120 g) salsa 12 (8-inch or 20 cm) whole grain tortillas
1 cup (245 g) hummus or 1 cup (240 ml)

Preparation

Drain from the sautéed vegetables some excess liquid. In a pan, add the peas, sautéed onions, sweet potatoes, nutritional yeast and salsa. Put it aside.

Using tortillas, hummus, bean mixture and 12 pieces of parchment paper or aluminum foil to set up an assembly line on the fridge.

Warm the tortillas one at a time. (Microwave them for about 15 seconds each, or bake them for 5 to 7 minutes at 350 ° F/180 ° C wrapped in a wet, lint-free towel.)

Lay hummus on a hot tortilla, then top with ½ cup (90 g) of bean-vegetable mixture. Roll, first pull the bottom and top in, then the sides in. Wrap the parchment or foil securely. Continue and top with the leftover tortillas. Enable cooling, then cooling for up to 5 days or freezing for up to 2 months.

Nutrition per serving: calorie: 200; Fat: 12g,; Carbohydrates: 63 g; Protein: 16 g

46. Veg Power-nuggets

Prep: 10 min (3 hours soaking lentils)
Cook Time: 20 min
Total: 30 min
Serves: 6

Ingredients

Lentils - 1 ½ cups
Carrot (sliced) - 1
Corn - ½ cup
Pea - ½ cup
Vegan cheddar cheese (shredded) - 1 cup

Dried oregano - 1 teaspoon
Salt - 1 teaspoon
Pepper - 1 teaspoon
Red pepper flakes - ½ teaspoon
Garlic - 1 clove

Preparation

Start by soaking the lentils for 3 hours in cold water.

Once the lentils are done soaking, set the temperature of the oven at 400 degrees Fahrenheit and let it preheat.

Take a baking tray and line it using parchment paper.

Now take a food processor and add in the carrots, peas, corn, vegan cheddar cheese, salt, oregano, pepper, garlic, soaked lentils and red pepper flakes. Pulse to mix all the ingredients well.

Form nuggets by taking 1 tablespoon of lentil mixture using your hands. Repeat the process with the rest of the mixture.

Place all the nuggets onto the lined baking tray. Bake for about 10 minutes. Flip over and bake for another 10 minutes.

Remove the baking tray from the oven and let the cutlets rest for about 5 minutes. Serve!

Nutrition per serving: Calories: 217 calories; Fat:7g; Carbohydrates:24 g; Protein:13g;

47. Tofu And Veggies Bulk-dha Bowl

Prep: 10 min
Cook Time: 40 min
Total: 50 min
Serves: 6

Ingredients

Sesame oil - 2 tablespoons
Sweet mirin - 2 tablespoons
Fiery Spice Blend - 1 tablespoon
Kosher salt - 1 teaspoon
Extra-firm tofu - 16 ounces
Sweet potatoes (rinse and peel) – 2 medium
Broccoli crowns - 2 medium
Quinoa (cooked) - 1 kg
Purple cabbage (thinly sliced) - 3 cups
English cucumber (julienned) - 3 cups
Avocado (thinly sliced) - 1 large

Peanuts (roasted) - ⅓ cup
Garnish
Fresh cilantro leaves – 1 tablespoon
Fresh mint leaf (torn) - 3 tablespoons
Fiery peanut sauce
Sesame oil - 2 tablespoons
Apple cider vinegar - 2 tablespoons
Fiery Spice Blend - 1 tablespoon
Cold water - ⅓ cup
Kosher salt – as per taste

Preparation

Start by preheating the oven by setting the temperature to 400 degrees Fahrenheit.

Now let us prepare the marinade for tofu. Take a medium-sized mixing bowl and add in the mirin, sesame oil, salt and fiery spice blend. Mix well.

Toss in the tofu cubes and mix well. Ensure all cubes are well coated. Cover it using a plastic wrap and place it in the refrigerator for about an hour.

Now take a large pot and fill it with cold water. Add salt and mix well. Toss in the sweet potatoes. Let it boil on medium-high flame.

Reduce the flame and let the sweet potatoes boil for 20 minutes.

Once done, remove the sweet potatoes from the water and set aside. In the same water, blanch the broccoli florets for about a minute and a half.

Remove the broccoli and add them to ice water. Let them sit in an ice bath for a minute. Remove and set aside on a plate lined with a paper towel. This will help in removing excess liquid.

Cut the boiled sweet potatoes lengthwise through the center. Further, cut into half-moon measuring 1 ½ -inch. Sprinkle with salt.

Take a baking sheet and grease it lightly. Place the sweet potato and marinated tofu onto the sheet.

Place it in the preheated oven and bake for about 20 minutes.

While the tofu and sweet potatoes are cooking. Let us prepare the fiery peanut sauce.

Take a medium mixing bowl and add in the apple cider vinegar, peanut butter, ¼ water and spice blend. Whisk well to combine.

Now, let us assemble the 6 tofu and veggies Buddha bowls. For this, in a bowl add 1 cup of quinoa, then follow it with 2 ½ ounces of tofu, ½ a cup of sweet potato, ½ a cup of broccoli, ½ a cup of purple cabbage, ½ a cup of cucumber and few slices of avocado.

Drizzle 2 tablespoons of peanut sauce and further top it with cilantro, mint and crushed peanuts.

Nutrition per serving: Calories: 957 calories; Fat:28g; Carbohydrates:144g; Protein: 39g

48. Crispy Tofu With Hoisin Sauce

Prep: 5 min
Cook Time: 15 min
Total: 20 min
Serves: 4

Ingredients

14 oz extra-firm tofu drained
½ tsp garlic powder
¼ tsp powdered ginger
½ tsp salt
¼ tsp pepper

1 tbsp peanut oil
1 tsp sesame oil
1 tbsp hoisin sauce

Preparation

To make this dish you need to first place your tofu in a fine-mesh strainer or colander and rinse. Set it aside.

In a bowl mix garlic powder, powdered ginger, salt and pepper together. Set it aside as well

Now cut the tofu into 1 inch cubes

Put a non-stick pan on the flame and add peanut oil and sesame oil and heat.

Now add the cubed tofu pieces into the pan and stir to coat with oil for about 5 minutes or until browned on one side

Sprinkle with your seasoning mix and stir until coated.

Continue cooking until all the sides are light-medium brown for about 10 to 15 minutes.

Pour hoisin sauce evenly onto the browned tofu pieces and stir until all the cubes are evenly coated with sauce.

Cook for 5 more minutes and wait until the tofu becomes dark brown and crispy. Remove from heat. You can serve it over stir-fried veggies or your favourite noodles and rice.

Per Serving: Calories: 106.3; Protein: 7g; Total fat: 18g; Carbohydrates: 3.4g; Fiber: 1g

49. Easy Chickpeas no-Meat-balls

Prep: 25 min
Cook Time: 1 hr
Total: 1 hr 25 min
Serves: 2

Ingredients

30g dried porcini mushrooms
3 tbsp olive oil
1 onion, very finely chopped
2 garlic cloves, crushed
1 tsp sweet smoked paprika
*1 x 400g can black beans, drained
and rinsed*
50g rolled oats
2 tbsp brown rice miso
50g fresh breadcrumbs
spaghetti or soft polenta, to serve

For the tomato sauce
2 tbsp olive oil
1 onion, very finely chopped
1 large garlic clove, crushed
Small pinch of chilli flakes
2 x 400g cans chopped tomatoes
1 tbsp soft brown sugar
*½ small bunch of basil, finely
chopped*

Preparation

Tip the dried porcini into a bowl, cover it with boiling water. Leave to soak for 20 minutes.

Heat 1 tbsp olive oil in a frying pan on a medium to high flame. Add onions and fry over a low heat for about 10 minutes or until it gets softened and translucent. Add the garlic and paprika and cook for 1 minute.

83

Now tip the black beans and oats into a food processor, continue until you have a chunky, textured mixture. Tip the beans into a mixing bowl and stir through the miso, breadcrumbs and cooked onion mix. Strain it. now finely chop the porcini mushrooms and add those. Make sure to not forget to keep the liquid for soup or risottos. Season and roll into 12 balls and chill in the fridge while you are preparing for the sauce.

Heat 2 tbsp oil in a saucepan, add the onion and fry over a low heat for about 10 minutes or until it get softened and translucent. Add the garlic and chilli and cook for at least 1 minute. Stir through the tomatoes and sugar, season to taste. Simmer uncovered for 20 minutes.

Now heat the oven to 180C/160C. Heat the remaining 2 tbsp oil for the meatballs in a nonstick fry pan over a medium flame. Add the balls and fry for 5 minutes on medium flame until they are evenly brown. Now transfer to a baking tray and put in the oven to cook for 12 minutes.

Add the cooked meatballs to a pan of sauce you made earlier, toss everything to coat then sprinkle the basil over it to give it a perfect flavor. Serve with spaghetti or soft polenta.

Per Serving: Calories: 400; Protein: 12g; Total fat: 17g; Carbohydrates: 45g; Fiber: 9

50. PAD THAI BOWL

Prep: 10 min
Cook Time: 10 min
Total: 20 min
Serves: 2

Ingredients

7 ounces brown rice noodles
1 teaspoon olive oil, or 1 tablespoon vegetable broth or water
2 carrots, peeled or scrubbed, and julienned
1 cup thinly sliced napa cabbage, or red cabbage
1 red bell pepper, seeded and thinly sliced
2 scallions, finely chopped

2 to 3 tablespoons fresh mint, finely chopped
1 cup bean sprouts
¼ cup Peanut Sauce
¼ cup fresh cilantro, finely chopped
2 tablespoons roasted peanuts, chopped
Fresh lime wedges

Preparation

Put the rice noodles in a large bowl or pot, and cover with boiling water. Let sit until they soften, about 10 minutes. Rinse, drain, and set aside to cool. Heat the oil in a large skillet to medium-high, and sauté the carrots, cabbage, and bell pepper until softened, 7 to 8 minutes. Toss in the scallions, mint, and bean sprouts and cook for just a minute or two, then remove from the heat.

Toss the noodles with the vegetables, and mix in the Peanut Sauce. Transfer to bowls, and sprinkle with cilantro and peanuts. Serve with a lime wedge to squeeze onto the dish for a flavor boost.

Per Serving; Calories: 660; Total fat: 19g; Carbs: 110g; Fiber: 10g; Protein: 15g

51. Green Pea Risotto

Prep: 5 min
Cook Time: 35 min
Total: 40 min
Serves: 4

Ingredients

1 teaspoon vegan butter
4 teaspoons minced garlic (about 4 cloves)
1 cup Arborio rice
2 cups vegetable broth
¼ teaspoon salt

2 tablespoons nutritional yeast
3 tablespoons lemon juice (about 1½ small lemons)
2 cups fresh, canned, or frozen (thawed) green peas
¼ to ½ teaspoon freshly ground black pepper, to taste

Preparation

In a large skillet over medium-high heat, heat the vegan butter.

Add the garlic and sauté for about 3 minutes.

Add the rice, broth, and salt, and stir to combine well.

Bring to boil. Reduce the heat to low and simmer for about 30 minutes, until the broth is absorbed and the rice is tender. Stir in the nutritional yeast and lemon juice.

Gently fold in the peas. Taste before seasoning with the pepper.

Divide the risotto evenly among 4 single-serving containers. Let cool before sealing the lids.

Place the containers in the refrigerator for up to 5 days.

Per Serving: Calories: 144; Fat: 2g; Protein: 10g; Carbohydrates: 24g; Fiber: 7g; Sugar: 5g; Sodium: 273mg

52. Hard Squat Salad

Prep: 10 min
Cook Time: 40 min
Total: 50 min
Serves: 4

Ingredients

3 medium golden beets
2 cups sliced sweet or Vidalia onions
1 teaspoon extra-virgin olive oil or no-beef broth

Pinch baking soda
¼ to ½ teaspoon salt, to taste
2 tablespoons unseasoned rice vinegar, white wine vinegar, or balsamic vinegar

Preparation

Cut the greens off the beets, and scrub the beets.

In a large pot, place a steamer basket and fill the pot with 2 inches of water.

Add the beets, bring to a boil, then reduce the heat to medium, cover, and steam for about 35 minutes, until you can easily pierce the middle of the beets with a knife.

Meanwhile, in a large, dry skillet over medium heat, sauté the onions for 5 minutes, stirring frequently.

Add the olive oil and baking soda, and continue cooking for 5 more minutes, stirring frequently. Stir in the salt to taste before removing from the heat. Transfer to a large bowl and set aside.

When the beets have cooked through, drain and cool until easy to handle. Rub the beets in a paper towel to easily remove the skins. Cut into wedges, and transfer to the bowl with the onions. Drizzle the vinegar over everything and toss well.

Divide the beets evenly among 4 wide-mouth jars or storage containers. Let cool before sealing the lids.

Per Serving: Calories: 104; Fat: 2g; Protein: 3g; Carbohydrates: 20g; Fiber: 4g; Sugar: 14g; Sodium: 303mg

53. Dig Deep Grilled Portobello

Prep: 20 min
Cook Time: 40 min
Total: 60 min
Serves: 4

Ingredients

4 *large portobello mushrooms*
1 *teaspoon olive oil*
Pinch sea salt
6 *large potatoes, scrubbed or peeled, and chopped*
3 *to 4 garlic cloves, minced*
½ *teaspoon olive oil*
½ *cup non-dairy milk*
2 *tablespoons coconut oil (optional)*

2 *cups green beans, cut into 1-inch pieces*
2 *to 3 teaspoons coconut oil*
2 *tablespoons nutritional yeast (optional)*
Pinch sea salt
Pinch sea salt
1 *to 2 tablespoons nutritional yeast (optional)*

Preparation

Preheat the grill to medium, or the oven to 350°F.

Take the stems out of the mushrooms.

Wipe the caps clean with a damp paper towel, then dry them. Spray the caps with a bit of olive oil, or put some oil in your hand and rub it over the mushrooms.

Rub the oil onto the top and bottom of each mushroom, then sprinkle them with a bit of salt on top and bottom.

Put the bottom side facing up on a baking sheet in the oven, or straight on the grill. They'll take about 30 minutes in the oven, or 20 minutes on the grill. Wait until they're soft and wrinkling around the edges. If you keep them bottom up, all the delicious mushroom juice will pool in the cap. Then at the very end, you can flip them over to drain the juice. If you like it, you can drizzle it over the mashed potatoes.

To Make The Mashed Potatoes:

Boil the chopped potatoes in lightly salted water for about 20 minutes, until soft. While they're cooking, sauté the garlic in the olive oil, or bake them whole in a 350°F oven for 10 minutes, then squeeze out the flesh.

Drain the potatoes, reserving about ½ cup water to mash them. In a large bowl, mash the potatoes with a little bit of the reserved water, the cooked garlic, milk, coconut oil (if using), nutritional yeast (if using), and salt to taste. Add more water, a little at a time, if needed, to get the texture

you want. If you use an immersion blender or beater to purée them, you'll have some extra-creamy potatoes .

To Make The Green Bean:

Heat a medium pot with a small amount of water to boil, then steam the green beans by either putting them directly in the pot or in a steaming basket.

Once they're slightly soft and vibrantly green, 7 to 8 minutes, take them off the heat and toss them with the oil, salt, and nutritional yeast (if using).

Per Serving: Calories: 263; Total fat: 7g; Carbs: 43g; Fiber: 7g; Protein: 10g

54. LENTIL SOUP

Prep: 10 min
Cook Time: 60 min
Total: 70 min
Serves: 4

Ingredients

2l veg stock
150g red lentils
6 carrots, finely chopped
2 medium leeks, sliced (300g)
Small handful chopped parsley, to serve

Preparation

Heat the stock in a large pan then add lentils in it. Give it a boil and allow the lentils to soften. If it's taking time, cook some more time.

Now add the carrots and leeks to the lentils and season salt. Make sure to not add salt if you're using ham stock because it will make it too salty. Let it boil, then reduce the heat, cover and simmer for 45 to 60 minutes until the lentils have broken down.

Scatter over the parsley and serve with buttered bread as per your choice.

Per Serving: Calories: 219; Protein: 12g; Total fat: 3g; Carbohydrates: 33g; Fiber: 9g

DINNERS

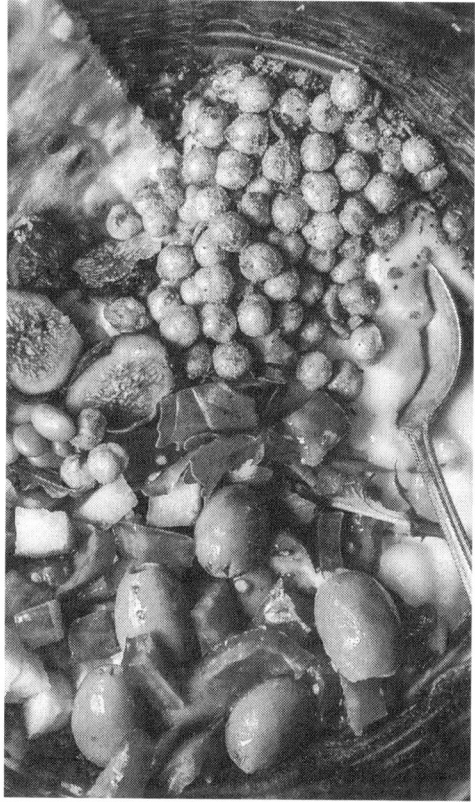

After a full day of working out and energy demanding life you need to recover nutrients. Particularly, you need to provide proteins to your body to elaborate them during the night.

55. Iron Abs Tabbouleh

Prep: 15 min
Cook Time: 10 min
Total: 25 min
Serves: 4

Ingredients

1 cup whole-wheat couscous
1 cup boiling water
Zest and juice of 1 lemon
1 garlic clove, pressed
Pinch of sea salt
1 tablespoon olive oil, or flaxseed oil (optional)

2 cups canned chickpeas
½ cucumber, diced small
1 tomato, diced small
1 cup fresh parsley, chopped
¼ cup fresh mint, finely chopped
2 scallions, finely chopped
4 tablespoons sunflower seeds

Preparation

Put the couscous in a medium bowl, and cover with boiling water until all the grains are submerged. Cover the bowl with a plate or wrap. Set aside.

Put the lemon zest and juice in a large salad bowl, then stir in the garlic, salt, and the olive oil (if using).

Put the cucumber, chickpeas, tomato, parsley, mint, and scallions in the bowl, and toss them to coat with the dressing. Take the plate off the couscous and fluff with a fork.

Add the cooked couscous to the vegetables, and toss to combine.

Serve topped with the sunflower seeds

Per Serving Calories: 304; Total fat: 11g; Carbs: 44g; Fiber: 6g; Protein: 10g

56. Mushroom Cream

Prep: 10 min
Cook Time: 20 min
Total: 30 min
Serves: 2

Ingredients

1 to 2 teaspoons olive oil
1 onion, chopped
2 garlic cloves, minced
2 cups chopped mushrooms
Pinch salt
2 tablespoons whole-grain flour

1 teaspoon dried herbs
4 cups Economical Vegetable Broth ,
store-bought broth, or water
1½ cups non dairy milk
Pinch freshly ground black pepper

Preparation

Heat the olive oil in a large soup pot over medium-high heat.

Add the onion, garlic, mushrooms, and salt. Sauté for about 5 minutes, until softened. Sprinkle the flour over the ingredients in the pot and toss to combine.

Cook for 1 to 2 minutes more to toast the flour.

Add the dried herbs, vegetable broth, milk, and pepper.

Turn the heat to low, and let the broth come to a simmer. (Don't bring to a full boil or the milk may separate.)

Cook for 10 minutes, until slightly thickened. Leftovers will keep in an airtight container for up to 1 week in the refrigerator or up to 1 month in the freezer.

Per Serving; Calories: 127; Protein: g; Total fat: 4g; Saturated fat: 0g; Carbohydrates: 21g; Fiber: 3g

57. CHINNING BAR TOFU SOUP

Prep: 40 min
Cook Time: 15 min
Total: 55 min
Serves: 3

Ingredients

6 to 7 ounces firm or extra-firm tofu
1 teaspoon olive oil
1 cup sliced mushrooms
1 cup finely chopped cabbage
1 garlic clove, minced
½-inch piece fresh ginger, peeled and minced
Salt

4 cups water or Vegetable Broth
2 tablespoons rice vinegar or apple cider vinegar
2 tablespoons soy sauce
1 teaspoon toasted sesame oil
1 teaspoon sugar
Pinch red pepper flakes
1 scallion, white and light green parts only, chopped

Preparation

Press your tofu before you start: Put it between several layers of paper towels and place a heavy pan or book (with a waterproof cover or protected with plastic wrap) on top. Let stand for 30 minutes. Discard the paper towels. Cut the tofu into ½-inch cubes.

In a large soup pot, heat the olive oil over medium-high heat.

Add the mushrooms, cabbage, garlic, ginger, and a pinch of salt. Sauté for 7 to 8 minutes, until the vegetables are softened.

Add the water, vinegar, soy sauce, sesame oil, sugar, red pepper flakes, and tofu.

Bring to a boil, then turn the heat to low. Simmer the soup for 5 to 10 minutes.

Serve with the scallion sprinkled on top.

Leftovers will keep in an airtight container for up to 1 week in the refrigerator or up to 1 month in the freezer.

Per Serving (2 cups): Calories: 161; Protein: 13g; Total fat: 9g; Saturated fat: 1g; Carbohydrates: 10g;

Fiber: 3g

58. FAST TWITCH QUINOA

Prep: 5 min
Cook Time: 0 min
Total: 5 min
Serves: 6-8

Ingredients

3 tablespoons olive oil
Juice of 1½ lemons
1 teaspoon garlic powder
½ teaspoon dried oregano
1 bunch curly kale, stemmed and roughly chopped
2 cups cooked tricolor quinoa

1 cup canned mandarin oranges in juice, drained
1 cup diced yellow summer squash
1 red bell pepper, seeded and diced
½ red onion, thinly sliced
½ cup dried cranberries or cherries
½ cup slivered almonds

Preparation

In a small bowl, whisk together the oil, lemon juice, garlic powder, and oregano.

In a large bowl, toss the kale with the oil-lemon mixture until well coated. Add the quinoa, oranges, squash, bell pepper, and red onion and toss until all the ingredients are well combined. Divide among bowls or transfer to a large serving platter. Top with the cranberries and almonds.

Per Serving (2 cups): Calories: 343; Protein: 24g; Total fat: 10.3g; Saturated fat: 1g; Carbohydrates: 109g; Fiber: 11g

59. Eggplant Parmesan

Prep: 10 min
Cook Time: 15 min
Total: 25 min
Serves: 1

Ingredients

¼ cup non dairy milk

¼ cup bread crumbs or panko

2 tablespoons nutritional yeast (optional)

¼ teaspoon salt

4 (¼-inch-thick) eggplant slices, peeled if desired

1 tablespoon olive oil, plus more as needed

4 tablespoons Simple Homemade Tomato Sauce

4 teaspoons Parm Sprinkle (vegan parmesan cheese)

Preparation

Put the milk in a shallow bowl. In another shallow bowl, stir together the bread crumbs, nutritional yeast (if using), and salt.

Dip one eggplant slice in the milk, making sure both sides get moistened. Dip it into the bread crumbs, flipping to coat both sides. Transfer to a plate and repeat to coat the remaining slices. Heat the olive oil in a large skillet over medium heat and add the breaded eggplant slices, making sure there is oil under each.

Cook for 5 to 7 minutes, until browned. Flip, adding more oil as needed. Top each slice with 1 tablespoon tomato sauce and 1 teaspoon Parm Sprinkle. Cook for 5 to 7 minutes more.

Per Serving Calories: 460; Protein: 9g; Total fat: 31g; Saturated fat: 4g; Carbohydrates: 31g; Fiber: 13g

60. APPLE-SUNFLOWER SPINACH SALAD

Prep: 5 min
Cook Time: 0 min
Total: 5 min
Serves: 1

Ingredients

1 cup baby spinach
½ apple, cored and chopped
¼ red onion, thinly sliced (optional)
2 tablespoons sunflower seeds or Cinnamon-Lime Sunflower Seeds

2 tablespoons dried cranberries
2 tablespoons Raspberry Vinaigrette
Canned cooked cannellini beans

Preparation

Arrange the spinach on a plate. Top with the apple, red onion (if using), cannellini beans, sunflower seeds, and cranberries, and drizzle with the vinaigrette.

Per Serving Calories: 444; Protein: 18.4g; Total fat: 28g; Saturated fat: 3g; Carbohydrates: 53g;

Fiber: 8g

61. Spaghetti Squash Primavera

Prep: 10 min
Cook Time: 40 min
Total: 50 min
Serves: 4

Ingredients

1 large spaghetti squash (roughly 4 pounds), halved and seeded
3 tablespoons olive oil, divided
1 onion, chopped
2 cups chopped broccoli florets
½ cup pitted and sliced green olives
1 cup halved cherry tomatoes
3 garlic cloves, minced

1½ teaspoons Italian seasoning
¾ teaspoon sea salt
½ teaspoon black pepper
1 cupDiced tofu
Pine nuts, for garnish (optional)
Walnut Parmesan or store-bought vegan Parmesan, for garnish (optional)
Red pepper flakes, for garnish (optional)

Preparation

Preheat the oven to 400°F. Line a baking sheet with parchment paper.

Brush the rims and the insides of both squash halves with 1 tablespoon of olive oil. Place on the prepared baking sheet, cut-sides down.

Bake for 35 to 45 minutes, until a fork can easily pierce the flesh. Set aside until cool enough to handle, 10 to 15 minutes.

At the same time, you can roast your tofu. Cube a block of tofu into your desired size, and sprinkle with salt and pepper. Place it in the oven alongside the squash and roast for 30-40 minutes, turning it halfway to get browning on both sides.

While the squash is cooling, heat 1 tablespoon of olive oil in a large skillet over medium heat.

Add the onion and broccoli and sauté for 3 minutes, or until the onion is soft. Add the olives and tomatoes and cook for an additional 3 to 5 minutes, until the broccoli is fork-tender and the tomatoes have started to wilt. Add the garlic and cook for 1 additional minute, or until fragrant. Remove from the heat. Use a fork to gently pull the squash flesh from the skin and separate the flesh into strands. The strands wrap around the squash horizontally, so rake your fork in the same direction as the strands to make the longest spaghetti squash noodles. Toss the noodles into the skillet with the vegetables. Add the final 1 tablespoon of olive oil, Italian seasoning, salt, and pepper and mix well to combine. Divide among bowls and garnish with pine nuts, Parmesan, and red pepper flakes, if desired.

Per Serving Calories: 200; Total fat: 1.1g; Carbs: 31.7g; Fiber: 7.2g; Protein: 19.4g

62. RED PEPPERS AND KALE

Prep: 5 min
Cook Time: 15 min
Total: 20 min
Serves: 4

Ingredients

2 cans (19 oz or 540ml each can) chickpeas (garbanzo beans) drained and rinsed
4 cloves garlic, minced
1 large sweet onion, chopped into long slices

4 tbsp olive oil
2 red peppers, chopped into long slices
6 cups kale, chopped into bite-sized pieces
Salt and pepper to taste

Preparation

Heat BBQ and prepare a greased BBQ basket or pan.

Meanwhile, mix together chickpeas, garlic, onion, red peppers and olive oil in a bowl and add to the BBQ basket and place on the grill. Stir regularly until chickpeas are slightly browned, onions and red peppers are softened and grilled.

When almost ready to serve add kale and stir constantly until the kale is slightly wilted. Serve immediately either on its own, or with garlic toast, pita bread or over rice.

Per Serving: Calories: 520; Total fat: 17g; Carbs: 78g; Fiber: 16g; Protein: 18g

63. CLEAN AND SNATCH SALAD

Prep: 5 min
Cook Time: 0 min
Total: 5 min
Serves: 4

Ingredients

1 (15.5-ounce) can chickpeas, drained and rinsed
1 (14-ounce) can hearts of palm, drained and chopped
½ cup chopped yellow or white onion
½ cup diced celery

¼ cup vegan mayonnaise, plus more if needed
½ teaspoon salt
¼ teaspoon freshly ground black pepper

Preparation

In a medium bowl, use a potato masher or fork to roughly mash the chickpeas until chunky and "shredded." Add the hearts of palm, onion, celery, vegan mayonnaise, salt, and pepper.

Combine and add more mayonnaise, if necessary, for a creamy texture. Into each of 4 single-serving containers, place ¾ cup of salad. Seal the lids.

Per Serving: Calories: 214; Fat: 6g; Protein: 9g; Carbohydrates: 35g; Fiber: 8g; Sugar: 1g; Sodium: 765mg

64. CAESAR PASTA

Prep: 10 min
Cook Time: 0 min
Total: 10 min
Serves: 1

Ingredients

2 cups chopped romaine lettuce
2 tablespoons Vegan Caesar Dressing
Vegan cheese, grated (optional)

½ cup cooked pasta
½ cup canned chickpeas, drained and rinsed
2 additional tablespoons Caesar Dressing

Preparation

In a large bowl, toss together the lettuce, dressing, and cheese (if using).

Add the pasta, chickpeas, and additional dressing. Toss to coat.

Per Serving: Calories: 415; Protein: 9g; Total fat: 8g; Saturated fat: 1g; Carbohydrates: 72g; Fiber: 13g

65. WARM POWER SALAD

Prep: 10 min
Cook Time: 15 min
Total: 25 min
Serves: 4

Ingredients

Salt for salting water, plus ¹/₂ teaspoon (optional)
4 red potatoes, quartered
1 pound carrots, sliced into ¹/₄-inch-thick rounds
1 tablespoon extra-virgin olive oil (optional)

2 tablespoons lime juice
2 teaspoons dried dill
¹/₄ teaspoon freshly ground black pepper
1 cup Cashew Cream or Parm-y Kale Pesto

Preparation

In a large pot, bring salted water to a boil. Add the potatoes and cook for 8 minutes. Add the carrots and continue to boil for another 8 minutes, until both the potatoes and carrots are crisp tender. Drain and return to the pot. Add the olive oil (if using), lime juice, dill, remaining ¹/₂ teaspoon of salt (if using), and pepper, and stir to coat well.

Divide the vegetables evenly among 4 single-compartment storage containers or wide-mouth pint glass jars, and spoon ¹/₄ cup of cream or pesto over the vegetables in each. Let cool before sealing the lids.

Per Serving: Calories: 393; Fat: 15g; Protein: 10g; Carbohydrates: 52g; Fiber: 9g; Sugar: 8g; Sodium: 343mg

66. CHEESE FREE MAC AND CHEESE

Prep: 10 min
Cook Time: 35 min
Total: 45 min
Serves: 2

Ingredient

For the tofu:
1/2 teaspoon garlic powder
2 tablespoons soy sauce
1 tablespoon cooking oil
1/4 teaspoon black salt
1 lb (450 g) firm tofu, chopped

For the cheese sauce: 2 teaspoons cornstarch
1 teaspoon red curry paste
1 cup (250 ml) almond milk
1 teaspoon garlic powder
1 1/2 cups (150 g) vegan cheddar cheese, shredded
To assemble:
8 oz (225 g) macaroni, uncooked
3 cups (150 g) baby spinach
1 cup (60 g) kale
Salt, to taste

Preparation

Combine the pepper, salt, garlic powder, oil, and soy sauce and in a bowl. Add the tofu and coat well.

Preheat a pan over medium heat. Add tofu and cook until browned on all sides.

Add water to a pot and bring to a boil. Add the macaroni and cook until tender.

Combine ½ cup milk with the cornstarch. Mix well until all the cornstarch has no lumps and is fully dissolved. Add the red curry paste and dissolve.

Add the remaining milk to the pot placed over medium heat, and add in the red curry slurry, vegan cheese and garlic powder. Stir thoroughly until the cheese has melted and the sauce is thick and smooth.

Add kale along with the spinach to the cooking pot with pasta, wilt it. Drain macaroni together with the greens and return the ingredients to the pot. Pour in the tofu and cheese sauce and stir to coat well.

Adjust on the seasonings as desired. Serve.

Per Serving: Calories: 376; Protein: 10g; Total fat: 16g; Carbohydrates: 47g; Fiber: 2g

67. Irish Stew

Prep: 10 min
Cook Time: 60 min
Total: 70 min
Serves: 4

Ingredients

½ cup Textured vegetable protein (TVP) chunks or soya chunks
Salt to taste
Pepper to taste
3 cloves garlic, minced
2 stalks celery, chopped
2 potatoes, peeled, chopped into chunks
1 ½ - 2 ½ cups vegetable stock

½ tablespoon minced fresh rosemary
2 tablespoons all-purpose flour
1 medium onion, chopped
1 cup button mushrooms or crimini mushrooms, halved or quartered depending on the size of the mushrooms
1 medium carrot, cut into thin, round slices
½ tablespoon minced, fresh thyme
1 tablespoon vegetable oil

Preparation

Add TVP into a bowl of hot water and let it soak for 30-40 minutes. Drain and set aside for 5-7 minutes.

Add flour, salt and pepper into a bowl and stir. Roll the TVP chunks in the flour mixture. Shake the chunks to drop off extra flour. Set aside the remaining flour mixture.

Place a soup pot over medium heat. Add 2 teaspoons oil and heat.

Add TVP and stir. Cook until brown all over.

Remove with a slotted spoon and place on a plate lined with paper towels.

Add ½ teaspoon oil into the pot. When the oil is heated, add garlic, salt, pepper and onion and sauté until onions are pink.

Add vegetables and herbs and mix well.

Add the retained flour mixture and sauté for 1-2 minutes.

Stir in the TVP stock. Stir constantly until it begins to boil.

Lower the heat and cover with a lid. Cook until tender. Stir occasionally.

Add more water or stock if you like to dilute the stew.

Season with salt and pepper.

Ladles into bowls and serve.

Per Serving: Calories: 229; Protein: 17.2g; Total fat: 4g; Carbohydrates: 10g; Fiber: 9.3g

68. QUIN-OTTO WITH DRIED TOMATOES

Prep: 10 min
Cook Time: 30 min
Total: 40 min
Serves: 2

Ingredients

3 cups vegetable broth

2 cloves garlic, minced
½ cup quinoa
¼ cup sun-dried tomatoes in oil, drained, sliced
1 teaspoon fresh chopped parsley
1 small onion, minced

1 ½ tablespoons olive oil
Salt to taste
Pepper to taste
2 tablespoons chopped fresh basil
3 tablespoons vegan parmesan cheese (optional)

Preparation

Place a saucepan over medium heat. Add oil. When the oil is heated, add onion and garlic and sauté until translucent.

Cook the quinoa: Cook 2/3 cup uncooked quinoa in water, according to package directions.

Add a cup of broth and mix well. Add salt and pepper to taste. Cook until nearly dry.

Add some more broth, tomatoes and herbs. Mix well. Cook until nearly dry.

Repeat adding the broth, a little at a time and cook until nearly dry each time, add cooked quinoa. Stir often.

Garnish with vegan Parmesan cheese and serve.

Per serving: Calories: 402; Fat: 13 g; Total Carbohydrates: 58 g; Fiber : 4 g; Protein: 11g

69. Steamed Eggplants With Peanut Dressing

Prep: 10 min
Cook Time: 20 min
Total: 30 min
Serves: 2

Ingredients:

6 ounces baby eggplants, halved lengthwise
½ tablespoon soy sauce
½ teaspoon sugar
1 teaspoon toasted sesame seeds
1 tablespoon chopped cilantro leaves, to garnish

1 tablespoon peanut butter
½ tablespoon rice vinegar
½ tablespoon chili oil + extra to serve
1 spring onion, thinly sliced
1 tablespoon boiling water

Preparation

Steam the eggplants in the steaming equipment you possess for about 15 minutes or until soft.

Place peanut butter in a bowl. Add boiling water into it and whisk well.

Add soy sauce, sugar, rice vinegar and chili oil and whisk well.

Place the eggplants on a serving platter. Trickle the sauce mixture over the eggplants.

Sprinkle sesame seeds, cilantro, spring onion on top. Drizzle some chili oil on top and serve.

Per Serving: Calories: 87; Protein: 3.8g; Total fat: 5.9g; Carbohydrates: 4.6g; Fiber: 2.9g

70. CAULIFLOWER RICE WOK

Prep: 10 min
Cook Time: 20 min
Total: 30 min
Serves: 4

Ingredients

1 lb (450 g) tofu
1/2 cup (150 g) peas, fresh or frozen 1
tablespoon ginger, minced
3 garlic cloves, minced
1/4 cup (30 g) green onions, sliced

1 cauliflower head, riced
2 carrots, diced
2 tablespoons sesame oil
3 tablespoons cashews
3 tablespoons soy sauce, or tamari sesame seeds, for garnish

Preparation

Press and drain the tofu. Then crumble it slightly in a bowl. Set aside.

Add oil to a wok pan and place over medium heat. Add the garlic and ginger and cook until slightly brown and fragrant, for about 1 minute. Add the tofu and stir for about 6 minutes, until golden and well cooked. Set the tofu aside.

Add more oil to the pan and add the carrots. Sauté for about 2-3 minutes until tender.

Add the peas along with the cauliflower rice and stir until combined. Cook for about 6-8 minutes, until the cauliflower becomes tender. Add the green onions, cooked tofu, cashews and soy sauce.

Serve the cauliflower fried rice and garnish with the sesame seeds. Enjoy!

Per Serving: Calories: 47; Protein: 2.14g; Total fat: 2.85g; Carbohydrates: 4.82g; Fiber: 3.2g

71. Spicy Root and Lentil Casserole

Prep: 10 min
Cook Time: 35 min
Total: 45 min
Serves: 4

Ingredients:

2 tbsp sunflower or vegetable oil
1 onion, chopped
2 garlic clove, crushed
700g potatoes, peeled and cut into chunks
4 carrot, thickly sliced
2 parsnip, thickly sliced
2 tbsp curry paste or powder
1 litre/1¾ pints vegetable stock

100g red lentils
a small bunch of fresh coriander, roughly chopped
low-fat yogurt
bread and naan bread, to serve

Preparation

Heat the oil in a large pan, cook the onion and garlic over a medium heat for 3 to 4 minutes or until they get softened. Continue stirring in between to cook them well. Add potatoes, carrots and parsnips, turn up the heat and cook for 6 to 7 minutes. keep stirring until the vegetables are golden.

Stir in the curry paste or powder, pour in the stock, bring to a boil. Reduce the heat, add the lentils. Cover and simmer for 15 to 20 minutes until the lentils and vegetables are tender and sauce has thickened.

Once done, season with coriander and heat for a minute. Top with yogurt and the rest of the coriander. If you wish you can have it with bread or naan

Per Serving: Calories: 378; Protein: 14g; Total fat: 9g; Carbohydrates: 64g; Fiber: 10g

72. COCONUT AND CURRY SOUP

Prep: 10 min
Cook Time: 20 min
Total: 30 min
Serves: 6

Ingredients

2½ cups red split lentils
2 cups onion, diced
2 cups carrots, diced
¾ cup frozen corn
¾ cup frozen peas
8 cups low sodium vegetable broth (2, 32oz.
cartons)
2 cups light coconut milk
1 tablespoon garam masala
1 tablespoon curry powder

½ teaspoon cayenne
1½ teaspoons sea salt
1 tablespoon vegetable oil
salt & pepper
chopped cilantro (optional)
cashew sour cream

Preparation

Heat oil in a large pot over medium-high heat. Add onions and sauté until softened and lightly browned, about 5 minutes. Add carrots, spices, and salt and sauté a few minutes more. Rinse lentils and add to the pot with coconut milk and vegetable broth. Bring to a boil then reduce to a simmer and cook covered for 15 minutes.

Transfer 2 cups of soup to a blender and puree. Return to the pot, add corn and peas, and simmer for 5 minutes more. Season with salt and pepper to taste.

Serve garnished with cashew sour cream and cilantro.

Nutrition per serving: Calories: 217.8 calories; Fat: 7.4g; Carbohydrates:28g; Protein: 11.1g

73. Free Weights Split Pea Soup

Prep: 10 min
Cook Time: 35 min
Total: 45 min
Serves: 6

Ingredients

3 or 4 carrots, scrubbed or peeled and chopped
1 large yellow onion, chopped
1 cup dried split green peas
3 cups water or unsalted vegetable broth
1 tablespoon tamari or soy sauce

2 to 3 teaspoons dried thyme or 1 teaspoon ground thyme
1 teaspoon onion powder
½ teaspoon garlic powder
Pinch freshly ground black pepper
¼ cup chopped sun-dried tomatoes or chopped pitted black olives
Salt

Preparation

Preparing the Ingredients. Combine the carrots, onion, split peas, water, tamari, thyme, onion powder, garlic powder, and pepper in your pot.

High pressure for 10 minutes . Close and lock the lid, then select High Pressure and set the time for 10 minutes.

Pressure Release . Let the pressure release naturally, about 20 minutes. Unlock and remove the lid. Let cool for a few minutes and then purée the soup—transfer the soup (in batches, if necessary) to a countertop blender.

Stir in the nutritional yeast (if using) and sun-dried tomatoes. Taste and season with salt.

Per Serving: Calories: 182; Protein: 12g; Total fat: 1g; Saturated fat: 11g; Carbohydrates: 26g; Fiber: 12g

74. CHICKPEA TOMATO SOUP

Prep: 10 min
Cook Time: 20 min
Total: 30 min
Serves: 2

Ingredients

1 to 2 teaspoons olive oil, or vegetable broth
½ cup chopped onion
3 garlic cloves, minced
1 cup mushrooms, chopped
⅛ to ¼ teaspoon sea salt, divided
1 tablespoon dried basil
½ tablespoon dried oregano

1 to 2 tablespoons balsamic vinegar, or red wine
1 (19-ounce) can diced tomatoes
1 (14-ounce) can chickpeas, drained and rinsed, or 1½ cups cooked
2 cups water
1 to 2 cups chopped kale

Preparation

In a large pot, warm the olive oil and sauté the onion, garlic, and mushrooms with a pinch of salt until softened, 7 to 8 minutes. Add the basil and oregano and stir to mix. Then add the vinegar to deglaze the pan, using a wooden spoon to scrape all the browned, savory bits up from the bottom. Add the tomatoes and chickpeas. Stir to combine, adding enough water to get the consistency you want. Add the kale and the remaining salt. Cover and simmer for 5 to 15 minutes, until the kale is as soft as you like it.

This is delicious topped with a tablespoon of toasted walnuts and a sprinkle of nutritional yeast, or the Cheesy Sprinkle.

Per Serving: Calories: 343; Protein: 17g; Total fat: 9g; Carbohydrates: 61g; Fiber: 15g

75. BEET AND SWEET POTATO SOUP

Prep: 10 min
Cook Time: 30 min
Total: 40 min
Serves: 6

Ingredients

5 cups water, or salt-free vegetable broth (if salted, omit the sea salt below)
1 to 2 teaspoons olive oil, or vegetable broth
1 cup chopped onion
3 garlic cloves, minced
1 tablespoon thyme, fresh or dried
1 to 2 teaspoons paprika
2 cups peeled and chopped beets

2 cups peeled and chopped sweet potato
2 cups peeled and chopped parsnips
½ teaspoon sea salt
1 cup fresh mint, chopped
½ avocado, or 2 tablespoons nut or seed butter (optional)
2 tablespoons balsamic vinegar (optional)
2 tablespoons pumpkin seeds

Preparation

In a large pot, boil the water. In another large pot, warm the olive oil and sauté the onion and garlic until softened, about 5 minutes.

Add the thyme, paprika, beets, sweet potato, and parsnips, along with the boiling water and salt.

Cover and leave to gently boil for about 30 minutes, or until the vegetables are soft.

Set aside a little mint for a garnish and add the rest, along with the avocado (if using).

Stir until well combined.

Transfer the soup to a blender or use an immersion blender to purée, adding the balsamic vinegar (if using).

Serve topped with fresh mint and pumpkin seeds—and maybe chunks of the other half of the avocado, if you used it. This soup is perfect to make in big batches and keep in single-serving containers in the freezer for quick weeknight meals.

Per Serving: Calories: 156; Protein: 9g; Total fat: 4g; Carbohydrates: 31g; Fiber: 7g

76. Dumbbell Kale Salad

Prep: 10 min
Cook Time: 20 min
Total: 30 min
Serves: 4

Ingredients

For the dressing:

1 avocado, peeled and pitted
1 tablespoon fresh lemon juice, or 1 teaspoon lemon juice concentrate and 2 teaspoons water
1 tablespoon fresh or dried dill
1 small garlic clove, pressed
1 scallion, chopped
Pinch sea salt
¼ cup water

For the salad:

8 large kale leaves
½ cup chopped green beans, raw or lightly steamed
1 cup cherry tomatoes, halved
1 bell pepper, chopped
2 scallions, chopped
2 cups cooked millet, or other cooked whole grain, such as quinoa or brown rice
Hummus (optional)

Preparation

To make the dressing:

Put all the ingredients in a blender or food processor. Purée until smooth, then add water as necessary to get the consistency you're looking for in your dressing. Taste for seasoning, and add more salt if you need to.

To make the salad:

Chop the kale, removing the stems if you want your salad less bitter, and then massage the leaves with your fingers until it wilts and gets a bit moist, about 2 minutes.

You can use a pinch of salt if you like to help it soften. Toss the kale with the green beans, cherry tomatoes, bell pepper, scallions, millet, and the dressing. Pile the salad onto plates, and top them off with a spoonful of hummus (if using).

Per Serving: Calories: 225; Total fat: 7g; Carbs: 37g; Fiber: 7g; Protein: 7g

77. Miso Noodle Soup

Prep: 10 min
Cook Time: 15 min
Total: 25 min
Serves: 4

Ingredients

7 ounces soba noodles (use 100% buckwheat for gluten-free)
4 cups water
4 tablespoons miso

1 cup adzuki beans (cooked or canned), drained and rinsed
2 tablespoons fresh cilantro, or basil, finely chopped
2 scallions, thinly sliced

Preparation

Bring a large pot of water to a boil, then add the soba noodles. Stir them occasionally; they'll take about 5 minutes to cook.

Meanwhile, prepare the rest of the soup by warming the water in a separate pot to just below boiling, then remove it from heat. Stir the miso into the water until it has dissolved. Once the soba noodles are cooked, drain them and rinse with hot water.

Add the cooked noodles, adzuki beans, cilantro, and scallions to the miso broth and serve.

Per Serving: Calories: 102; Protein: 11g; Total fat: 1g; Saturated fat: 11g; Carbohydrates: 18g; Fiber: 5g

78. Creamy Butternut Squash Soup

Prep: 10 min
Cook Time: 35 min
Total: 45 min
Serves: 4-6

Ingredients

2 tablespoons olive oil or 1/4 cup water (for water saute)
1 medium yellow onion, diced
1 large butternut squash, cubed (about 8 cups)

1 1/2 cups orange lentils
2 teaspoons dried sage or 2 tablespoons fresh minced
7 cups vegetable broth or water (or combo)
mineral salt & white or fresh cracked pepper, to taste

Preparation

In a large stockpot, combine the squash, bell pepper, onion, garlic, orange lentil and broth.

Mix well to combine, cover, and bring to a boil.

Reduce to a simmer and cook, covered, for 15 minutes, or until the squash is fork-tender. Add the lemon juice, maple syrup, salt, and pepper and stir well to combine.

Carefully transfer the soup to a blender. Remove the plug from the blender lid to allow steam to escape, hold a towel firmly over the hole in the lid, and blend until smooth.

Start on the lowest speed possible and increase gradually until the soup is completely smooth. Depending on your blender capacity, this might have to be done in two batches. (If you have an immersion blender, it would work great here.) Gently reheat over a low heat to serve.

Per Serving Calories: 421; Total fat: 4.5g; Carbs: 81.1g; Fiber: 13.9g; Protein: 20.9g

79. SEITAN

Prep: 25 min
Cook Time: 20 min
Total: 45 min
Serves: 4-6

Ingredients

Firm Tofu, 250 gram
Unsweetened soy milk, 150ml
Miso paste 2 tsp
Marmite 2 tsp
Onion powder 1 tsp
Garlic powder 2 tsp

Wheat gluten 160g
Pea protein or vegan protein powder, 40g
Vegetable stock 1 ½ litres

Preparation

Blitz the tofu, soy milk, miso, marmite, onion powder, garlic powder, 1 tsp salt and ½ tsp white pepper in a food processor. Blend until smooth.

Tip into a bowl and add the wheat gluten and pea protein or protein powder. Mix them all to form a dough. Knead the dough well, stretching and tearing for 10-15 minutes. you'll feel it ready once the dough feels springy.

Pour the vegetable stock into a pan and let it simmer. Flatten out the seitan to a thickness of 1 cm and chop into chicken-breast-sized chunks. Simmer it in the stock for 20 minutes covering with a lid. Once it's done, allow it to cool down. The best way is to do this the day before and leave to chill in the fridge. The seitan chunks can also be frozen if you wish. When you're ready to use the seitan in a recipe—just pat it dry with kitchen paper. Chop or tear it into smaller pieces before cooking as per your choice.

Per Serving: Calories: 211; Protein: 35g; Total fat: 5g; Carbohydrates: 6g; Fiber: 2g

Try it with broccoli, red bell pepper and scallions. Simply fry the seitan chunks in a pan or skillet with some oil and soy sauce for 5 minutes. Remove it and put it aside. Use the same pan for frying broccoli, bell pepper and scallions with a bit of water for 3 minutes. Put your seitan chunks back into the pan and stir everything together for one minute or two. Just add some teriyaki sauce at the end.

80. TOFU KUMQUAT RADISH SALAD

Prep: 10 min
Cook Time: 5 min
Total: 15 min
Serves: 2

Ingredients:

200g firm tofu
2 tbsp sesame seeds
1 tbsp Japanese shichimi togarashi spice mix
½ tbsp cornflour
1 tbsp sesame oil
1 tbsp vegetable oil

200g Tenderstem broccoli
100g sugar snap peas
4 radishes, thinly sliced
2 spring onions, finely chopped
3 kumquats, thinly sliced

For the dressing

2 tbsp low-salt Japanese soy sauce
2 tbsp Yuzu juice (or 1 tbsp each lime and grapefruit juice)
1 tsp golden caster sugar
1 small shallot, finely diced

Preparations

Slice the tofu in half, wrap well in kitchen paper and put on a plate. Place a heavy fry pan on top to squeeze the water out of it. Set it aside. Change the paper a few times until the tofu feels dry. Once it's done cut it into chunky slices.

Mix together the sesame seeds, Japanese spice mix and cornflour in a bowl. Sprinkle over the tofu until well coated. Set aside.

Take a small bowl, mix the dressing ingredients together and set aside. Bring a pan of water to the boil for the vegetables. Now heat the sesame oil and vegetable oil in a large frying pan.

Once the oils get heated up add tofu and fry for 1 minute or until the both sides are nicely browned in color. Repeat the same procedure with the remaining tofu.

Now in the boiled water, cook the broccoli and sugar snap peas for 2 to 3 minutes. Drain and divide between two large shallow bowls. Top with the tofu and drizzle over the dressing.

Scatter the radishes, spring onions and kumquats on top.

Per Serving
Calories: 528; Protein: 27g; Total fat: 33g; Carbohydrates: 24g; Fiber: 12g

DESSERTS

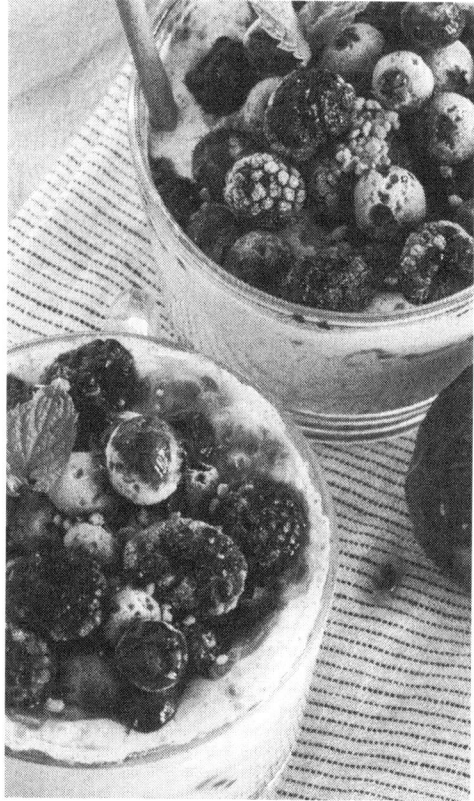

No pain no gain.

Ok, right, but you can enjoy some sweet treat every now and then, as long as it fits your macros.

81. ZESTY ORANGE-CRANBERRY ENERGY BITES

Prep: 10 min
Cook Time: 15 min
Total: 25 min
Serves: 12 bites

Ingredients

2 tablespoons almond butter, or cashew or sunflower seed butter
2 tablespoons maple syrup, or brown rice syrup
¾ cup cooked quinoa
¼ cup sesame seeds, toasted

1 tablespoon chia seeds
½ teaspoon almond extract, or vanilla extract
Zest of 1 orange
1 tablespoon dried cranberries
¼ cup ground almonds

Preparation

In a medium bowl, mix together the nut or seed butter and syrup until smooth and creamy. Stir in the rest of the ingredients, and mix to make sure the consistency is holding together in a ball. Form the mix into 12 balls.

Place them on a baking sheet lined with parchment or waxed paper and put in the fridge to set for about 15 minutes.

If the balls aren't holding together, it's likely because of the moisture content of your cooked quinoa. Add more nut or seed butter mixed with syrup until it all sticks together.

Per Serving (1 bite): Calories: 109; Total fat: 7g; Carbs: 11g; Fiber: 3g; Protein: 3g

82. BANANA-NUT BREAD BARS

Prep: 5 min
Cook Time: 30 min
Total: 35 min
Serves: 9

Ingredients

Nonstick cooking spray (optional)
2 large ripe bananas
1 tablespoon maple syrup
½ teaspoon vanilla extract

2 cups old-fashioned rolled oats
½ teaspoons salt
¼ cup chopped walnuts

Preparation

Preheat the oven to 350°F. Lightly coat a 9-by-9-inch baking pan with nonstick cooking spray (if using) or line with parchment paper for oil-free baking.

In a medium bowl, mash the bananas with a fork. Add the maple syrup and vanilla extract and mix well. Add the oats, salt, and walnuts, mixing well.

Transfer the batter to the baking pan and bake for 25 to 30 minutes, until the top is crispy. Cool completely before slicing into 9 bars.

Transfer to an airtight storage container or a large plastic bag.

Per Serving (1 bar): Calories: 73; Protein: 2g; Total fat: 1g; Carbohydrates: 15g; Fiber: 2g

83. APPLE CRUMBLE

Prep: 20 min
Cook Time: 25 min
Total: 45 min
Serves: 6

Ingredients

For The Filling

4 to 5 apples, cored and chopped (about 6 cups)
½ cup unsweetened applesauce, or ¼ cup water
2 to 3 tablespoons unrefined sugar (coconut, date, sucanat, maple syrup)
1 teaspoon ground cinnamon
Pinch sea salt

For The Crumble

2 tablespoons almond butter, or cashew or sunflower seed butter
2 tablespoons maple syrup
1½ cups rolled oats
½ cup walnuts, finely chopped
½ teaspoon ground cinnamon
2 to 3 tablespoons unrefined granular sugar (coconut, date, sucanat)

Preparation

Preheat the oven to 350°F. Put the apples and applesauce in an 8-inch-square baking dish, and sprinkle with the sugar, cinnamon, and salt. Toss to combine.

In a medium bowl, mix together the nut butter and maple syrup until smooth and creamy.

Add the oats, walnuts, cinnamon, and sugar and stir to coat, using your hands if necessary. (If you have a small food processor, pulse the oats and walnuts together before adding them to the mix.)

Sprinkle the topping over the apples, and put the dish in the oven.

Bake for 20 to 25 minutes, or until the fruit is soft and the topping is lightly browned.

Per Serving: Calories: 356; Protein: 7g; Total fat: 17g; Carbohydrates: 49g; Fiber: 7g

84. CASHEW-CHOCOLATE TRUFFLES

Prep: 15 min
Cook Time: 0 min
Total: 15 min
Serves: 12

Ingredients

1 cup raw cashews, soaked in water overnight
¾ cup pitted dates
2 tablespoons coconut oil

1 cup unsweetened shredded coconut, divided
1 to 2 tablespoons cocoa powder, to taste

Preparation

In a food processor, combine the cashews, dates, coconut oil, ½ cup of shredded coconut, and cocoa powder. Pulse until fully incorporated; it will resemble chunky cookie dough. Spread the remaining ½ cup of shredded coconut on a plate.

Form the mixture into tablespoon-size balls and roll on the plate to cover with the shredded coconut. Transfer to a parchment paper–lined plate or baking sheet. Repeat to make 12 truffles.

Place the truffles in the refrigerator for 1 hour to set. Transfer the truffles to a storage container or freezer-safe bag and seal.

Per Serving: Calories: 238; Protein: 3g; Total fat: 18g; Carbohydrates: 16g; Fiber: 4g

85. BANANA CHOCOLATE CUPCAKES

Prep: 20 min
Cook Time: 20 min
Total: 40 min
Serves: 12

Ingredients

3 medium bananas
1 cup non-dairy milk
2 tablespoons almond butter
1 teaspoon apple cider vinegar
1 teaspoon pure vanilla extract
1 ¼ cups whole-grain flour
½ cup rolled oats

¼ cup coconut sugar (optional)
1 teaspoon baking powder
½ teaspoon baking soda
½ cup unsweetened cocoa powder
¼ cup chia seeds, or sesame seeds
Pinch sea salt
¼ cup dark chocolate chips, dried cranberries, or raisins (optional)

Preparation

Preheat the oven to 350°F. Lightly grease the cups of two 6-cup muffin tins or line with paper muffin cups.

Put the bananas, milk, almond butter, vinegar, and vanilla in a blender and purée until smooth.

Or stir together in a large bowl until smooth and creamy.

Put the flour, oats, sugar (if using), baking powder, baking soda, cocoa powder, chia seeds, salt, and chocolate chips in another large bowl, and stir to combine.

Mix together the wet and dry ingredients, stirring as little as possible. Spoon into muffin cups, and bake for 20 to 25 minutes. Take the cupcakes out of the oven and let them cool fully before taking out of the muffin tins, since they'll be very moist.

Per Serving(1 cupcake): Calories: 215; Protein: 6g; Total fat: 6g; Carbohydrates: 39g; Fiber: 9g

86. MINTY FRUIT SALAD

Prep: 15 min
Cook Time: 20 min
Total: 35 min
Serves: 8

Ingredients

2/3 cup uncooked white quinoa (or 2 cups cooked quinoa)
1/4 cup chopped mint, loosely packed
juice of 1 lime (about 3 tablespoons)
2 tablespoons honey
2 cups strawberries, quartered

1 cup blueberries
1 cup kiwi, peeled and chopped
15 ounce can mandarins, drained (no sugar added; OR use 3–4 small fresh mandarins)
2 bright yellow bananas, peeled and sliced

Preparation

Cook the quinoa: Cook 2/3 cup uncooked quinoa in water, according to package directions. You can also use 2 cups of precooked quinoa.

Make the dressing: In a small bowl, whisk mint, lime juice and honey until well mixed.

Put it together: In a large bowl, combine cooked quinoa with all the fruit (strawberries, blueberries, kiwi, mandarins & bananas), then pour the dressing over the top and combine until well mixed. Serve immediately, or prepare up to 6 hours in advance for best appearance.

Storage: The leftovers will keep for up to 4 days; however the strawberries will start to bleed into the quinoa and the bananas will get a bit mushy, but it will still taste good.

Per Serving: Calories: 171; Fat: 1g; Protein: 4g; Carbohydrates: 39g; Fiber: 6g; Sugar: 22g; Sodium: 6mg

87. Mango Coconut Cream Pie

Prep: 20 min
Chill Time: 30 min
Total: 50 min
Serves: 8

Ingredients

For the crust

½ *cup rolled oats*
1 *cup cashews*
1 *cup soft pitted dates*

For the filling

1 *cup canned coconut milk*
½ *cup water*
2 *large mangos, peeled and chopped, or about 2 cups frozen chunks*
½ *cup unsweetened shredded coconut*

Preparation

Put all the crust ingredients in a food processor and pulse until it holds together.

If you don't have a food processor, chop everything as finely as possible and use ½ cup cashew or almond butter in place of half the cashews.

Press the mixture down firmly into an 8-inch pie or springform pan.

Put the all filling ingredients in a blender and purée until smooth (about 1 minute). It should be very thick, so you may have to stop and stir until it's smooth.

Pour the filling into the crust, use a rubber spatula to smooth the top, and put the pie in the freezer until set, about 30 minutes. Once frozen, it should be set out for about 15 minutes to soften before serving.

Top with a batch of *Coconut Whipped Cream* scooped on top of the pie once it's set. Finish it off with a sprinkling of toasted shredded coconut.

Per Serving (1 slice): Calories: 427; Total fat: 28g; Carbs: 45g; Fiber: 6g; Protein: 8g

88. CHERRY-VANILLA RICE PUDDING

Prep: 5 min
Cook Time: 55 min
Total: 1 hour
Serves: 4-6

Ingredients

1 cup short-grain brown rice
1¾ cups non dairy milk, plus more as needed
1½ cups water
4 tablespoons unrefined sugar or pure maple syrup (use 2 tablespoons if you use a sweetened milk), plus more as needed

1 teaspoon vanilla extract (use ½ teaspoon if you use vanilla milk)
Pinch salt
¼ cup dried cherries or ½ cup fresh or frozen pitted cherries

Preparation

Preparing the Ingredients. In your electric pressure cooker's cooking pot, combine the rice, milk, water, sugar, vanilla, and salt.

High pressure for 30 minutes. Close and lock the lid, and select High Pressure for 30 minutes.

Pressure Release. Once the cook time is complete, let the pressure release naturally, about 20 minutes. Unlock and remove the lid. Stir in the cherries and put the lid back on loosely for about 10 minutes. Serve, adding more milk or sugar, as desired.

Per Serving: Calories: 177; Total fat: 1g; Protein: 3g; Sodium: 27mg; Fiber: 2g

89. LIME IN THE COCONUT CHIA PUDDING

Prep: 10 min
Chill Time: 20 min
Total: 30 min
Serves: 4

Ingredients

Zest and juice of 1 lime
1 (14-ounce) can coconut milk
1 to 2 dates, or 1 tablespoon coconut or other unrefined sugar, or 1 tablespoon maple syrup, or 10 to 15 drops pure liquid stevia

2 tablespoons chia seeds, whole or ground
2 teaspoons matcha green tea powder (optional)

Preparation

Blend all the ingredients in a blender until smooth. Chill in the fridge for about 20 minutes, then serve topped with one or more of the topping ideas.

Try blueberries, blackberries, sliced strawberries, Coconut Whipped Cream, or toasted unsweetened coconut.

Per Serving: Calories : 226; Total fat: 20g; Carbs: 13g; Fiber: 5g; Protein: 3g

90. Mint Chocolate Chip Sorbet

Prep: 5 min
Cook Time: 0 min
Total: 5 min
Serves: 1

Ingredients

1 frozen banana
1 tablespoon almond butter, or peanut butter, or other nut or seed butter
2 tablespoons fresh mint, minced

¼ cup or less non-dairy milk (only if needed)
2 to 3 tablespoons non-dairy chocolate chips, or cocoa nibs
2 to 3 tablespoons goji berries (optional)

Preparation

Put the banana, almond butter, and mint in a food processor or blender and purée until smooth.

Add the non-dairy milk if needed to keep blending (but only if needed, as this will make the texture less solid). Pulse the chocolate chips and goji berries (if using) into the mix so they're roughly chopped up.

Per Serving: Calories: 212; Total fat: 10g; Carbs: 31g; Fiber: 4g; Protein: 3g

91. PEACH-MANGO CRUMBLE

Prep: 10 min
Cook Time: 11 min
Total: 21 min
Serves: 4-6

Ingredients

3 cups chopped fresh or frozen peaches
3 cups chopped fresh or frozen mangos
4 tablespoons unrefined sugar or pure maple syrup, divided
1 cup gluten-free rolled oats
½ cup shredded coconut, sweetened or unsweetened
2 tablespoons coconut oil or vegan margarine

Preparation

In a 6- to 7-inch round baking dish, toss together the peaches, mangos, and 2 tablespoons of sugar.

In a food processor, combine the oats, coconut, coconut oil, and remaining 2 tablespoons of sugar.

Pulse until combined. (If you use maple syrup, you'll need less coconut oil. Start with just the syrup and add oil if the mixture isn't sticking together.) Sprinkle the oat mixture over the fruit mixture.

Cover the dish with aluminum foil. Put a trivet in the bottom of your electric pressure cooker's cooking pot and pour in a cup or two of water. Using a foil sling or silicone helper handles, lower the pan onto the trivet.

High pressure for 6 minutes. Close and lock the lid, and select High Pressure for 6 minutes.

Pressure Release. Once the cooking time is complete, quickly release the pressure. Unlock and remove the lid.

Let cool for a few minutes before carefully lifting out the dish with oven mitts or tongs. Scoop out portions to serve.

Per Serving: Calories: 321; Total fat: 18g; Protein: 4g; Sodium: 2mg; Fiber: 7g

Smoothies

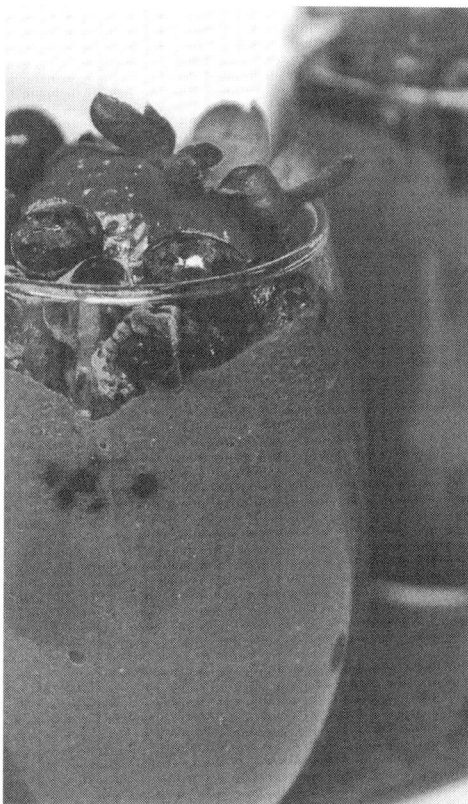

Smoothies are the best.

Quick to prepare, quick to consume, and you can add the vegan supplements you need according to your training phase.

92. BERRY PROTEIN SMOOTHIE

Prep: 5 min
Cook Time: 0 min
Total: 5 min
Serves: 1

Ingredients

1 banana
1 cup fresh or frozen berries
¾ cup water or non dairy milk, plus more as needed
1 scoop plant-based protein powder, 3 ounces silken tofu, ¼ cup rolled oats, or ½ cup cooked quinoa

Additions
1 tablespoon ground flaxseed or chia seeds
1 handful fresh spinach or lettuce, or 1 chunk cucumber
Coconut water to replace some of the liquid

Preparation

In a blender, combine the banana, berries, water, and your choice of protein.

Add any additional ingredients as desired. Purée until smooth and creamy, about 50 seconds.

Add a bit more water if you like a thinner smoothie.

Per Serving: Calories: 332; Protein: 7g; Total fat: 5g; Saturated fat: 1g; Carbohydrates: 72g; Fiber: 11g

93. GREEN KICKSTART SMOOTHIE

Prep: 5 min
Cook Time: 0 min
Total: 5 min
Serves: 1

Ingredients

½ avocado or 1 banana
½ cup chopped cucumber, peeled if desired
1 handful fresh spinach or chopped lettuce
1 pear or apple, peeled and cored, or 1 cup
unsweetened applesauce
2 tablespoons freshly squeezed lime juice
1 cup water or non dairy milk, plus more as
needed

Additions
½-inch piece peeled fresh ginger
1 tablespoon ground flaxseed or chia
seeds
½ cup soy yogurt or 3 ounces silken tofu
Coconut water to replace some of the
liquid
2 tablespoons chopped fresh mint or ½
cup chopped mango

Preparation

In a blender, combine the avocado, cucumber, spinach, pear, lime juice, and
water.

Add any Additions ingredients as desired. Purée until smooth and creamy, about
50 seconds. Add a bit more water if you like a thinner smoothie.

Per Serving: Calories: 263; Protein: 4g; Total fat: 14g; Saturated fat: 2g; Carbohydrates: 36g; Fiber:

10g

94. MANGO KEY LIME PIE SMOOTHIE

Prep: 5 min
Cook Time: 0 min
Total: 5 min
Serves: 1

Ingredients

¼ avocado
1 cup baby spinach
½ cup frozen mango chunks

1 cup unsweetened soy or almond milk
Juice of 1 lime (preferably a Key lime).
1 tablespoon maple syrup

Preparation

Combine all the ingredients in a blender and blend until smooth. Enjoy immediately.

Per Serving: Calories: 620; Protein: 11g; Total fat: 27g; Saturated fat: 16g; Carbohydrates: 85g; Fiber: 2g

95. BLUEBERRY LEMONADE SMOOTHIE

Prep: 5 min
Cook Time: 0 min
Total: 5 min
Serves: 1

Ingredients

1 cup roughly chopped kale
¾ cup frozen blueberries
1 cup unsweetened soy or almond milk
Juice of 1 lemon
1 tablespoon maple syrup

Preparation

Combine all the ingredients in a blender and blend until smooth. Enjoy immediately.

Per Serving: Calories: 190; Protein: 1g; Total fat: 0g; Carbohydrates: 44g; Fiber: 3g

96. GREAT GREEN SMOOTHIE

Prep: 5 min
Cook Time: 0 min
Total: 5 min
Serves: 4

Ingredients

4 bananas, peeled
4 cups hulled strawberries
4 cups spinach
4 cups plant-based milk

Preparation

Open 4 quart-size, freezer-safe bags. In each, layer in the following order: 1 banana (halved or sliced), 1 cup of strawberries, and 1 cup of spinach. Seal and place in the freezer.

To serve, take a frozen bag of Great Green Smoothie ingredients and transfer to a blender. Add 1 cup of plant-based milk, and blend until smooth. Place freezer bags in the freezer for up to 2 months.

Per Serving: Calories: 173; Protein: 4g; Total fat: 2g; Carbohydrates: 40g; Fiber: 7g

97. Chocolate Peanut Butter Smoothie

Prep: 5 min
Cook Time: 0 min
Total: 5 min
Serves: 1 cup

Ingredients

Water as needed
2 tbsp flax meal
1 tbsp unsweetened cocoa powder

1 tbsp natural peanut butter
1 scoop chocolate whey protein powder

Preparations

Preparing the Ingredients

In a blender, add water, unsweetened cocoa powder, natural peanut butter, 1 scoop chocolate whey protein powder, and flax meal. Puree until smooth and creamy.

Add a bit more water if you like thinner consistency

Per Serving: Calories: 347; Protein: 33g; Total fat: 17g; Carbohydrates: 19g; Fiber: 9g

98. CHOCOLATE **PB** SMOOTHIE

Prep: 5 min
Cook Time: 0 min
Total: 5 min
Serves: 4

Ingredients

1 banana
¼ cup rolled oats, or 1 scoop plant protein powder
1 tablespoon flaxseed, or chia seeds
1 tablespoon unsweetened cocoa powder
1 tablespoon peanut butter, or almond or sunflower seed butter

1 tablespoon maple syrup (optional)
1 cup alfalfa sprouts, or spinach, chopped (optional)
½ cup non-dairy milk (optional)
1 cup water
OPTIONAL
1 teaspoon matcha powder
1 teaspoon cocoa nibs

Preparation

Purée everything in a blender until smooth, adding more water (or non-dairy milk) if needed. Add bonus boosters, as desired. Purée until blended.

Per Serving: Calories: 474; Protein: 13g; Total fat: 16g; Carbohydrates: 79g; Fiber: 18g

99. BERRY PROTEIN SMOOTHIE

Prep: 5 min
Cook Time: 0 min
Total: 5 min
Serves: 1

Ingredients

1 banana
1 cup fresh or frozen berries
¾ cup water or non dairy milk, plus more if needed
1 scoop plant-based protein powder, 3 ounces silken tofu, ¼ cup rolled oats, or ½ cup cooked quinoa

1 tablespoon ground flaxseed or chia seeds
1 handful fresh spinach or lettuce, or 1 chunk cucumber
Coconut water to replace some of the liquid

Preparation

In a blender, combine the banana, berries, water, and your choice of protein.

Add any additional ingredients as desired. Purée until smooth and creamy, about 50 seconds.

Add a bit more water if you like a thinner smoothie.

Per Serving: Calories: 332; Protein: 7g; Total fat: 5g; Saturated fat: 1g; Carbohydrates: 72g; Fiber: 11g

100. BLUEBERRY AND CHIA SMOOTHIE

Prep: 10 min
Cook Time: 0 min
Total: 10 min
Serves: 2

Ingredients

2 tablespoons chia seeds
2 cups unsweetened non dairy milk
2 cups blueberries, fresh or frozen

2 tablespoons pure maple syrup or agave
2 tablespoons cocoa powder

Preparation

Soak the chia seeds in the almond milk for 5 minutes.

In a blender, combine the soaked chia seeds, almond milk, blueberries, maple syrup, and cocoa powder and blend until smooth. Serve immediately.

Per Serving: Calories: 283; Protein: 7g; Total fat: 8g; Saturated fat: 1g; Carbohydrates: 54g; Fiber: 12g

101. Pink Panther Smoothie

Prep: 5 min
Cook Time: 0 min
Total: 5 min
Serves: 3 cups

Ingredients

1 cup strawberries
1 cup chopped melon (any kind)
1 cup cranberries, or raspberries
1 tablespoon chia seeds
½ cup coconut milk, or other non-dairy milk
1 cup water

(OPTIONAL)
1 teaspoon goji berries
2 tablespoons fresh mint, chopped

Preparation

Purée everything in a blender until smooth, adding more water (or coconut milk) if needed.

Add bonus boosters, as desired. Purée until blended. If you don't have (or don't like) coconut, try using sunflower seeds for an immune boost of zinc and selenium.

Per Serving (3 Cups) : Calories: 459; Protein: 8g; Total fat: 30g; Carbohydrates: 52g; Fiber: 19g

Four Week Plan

The following is just an example of a possible 4 week meal high protein vegan plan.

Of course this is not a "one plan fits all", since no such thing as a one plan fits all exists when it comes to designing the ideal diet for a bodybuilder workout schedule.

A lot of variables must be considered, such as the phase of training you are at, your body type and metabolism, the intensity and frequency of your training and so on.

This Meal Plan is mainly intended to give you an idea of a variated, healthy and macros balanced, high protein diet, that can successfully backup an intense bodybuilding training plan. And delicious too, which never hurts.

Most of the recipes contain both protein, fat and carbs, then it's up to you to adapt the macros balancing according to your specific situation (and taste, of course).

Now, before I leave you with the Four Week Plan, I want to thank you for purchasing this book, but even more for deciding to put yourself in the middle of this challenge that is growing muscle and strength with intense training relying only on plant based food.

Whatever is the reason that brought you on this path, you are doing the right thing and you have all my respect.

This book was just intended as a cookbook with some ideas for vegan high protein recipes, that you can follow or adapt as you need or prefer.

Many of you are readers of my previous book *The Vegan Bodybuilder*, you may even be among the ones that asked me to write a cookbook after reading that one.

But if you just bumped into this one when looking for some vegan cookbook for athletes, you may be interested in reading a little about the theories behind green fuel for the athletes, or knowing some more about properties and benefits of different vegan foods.

If that's the case I'd be more than happy if you would consider my *The Vegan Bodybuilder*.

And of course, I would be happy to get some feedback from you, if you'd like to.

I love compliments (who doesn't) but I equally love insights on what I could have done better. So please feel free to have your say in my inbox at zhnardella@gmail.com.

I'll be happy to hear from you, and I always try to reply to any message.

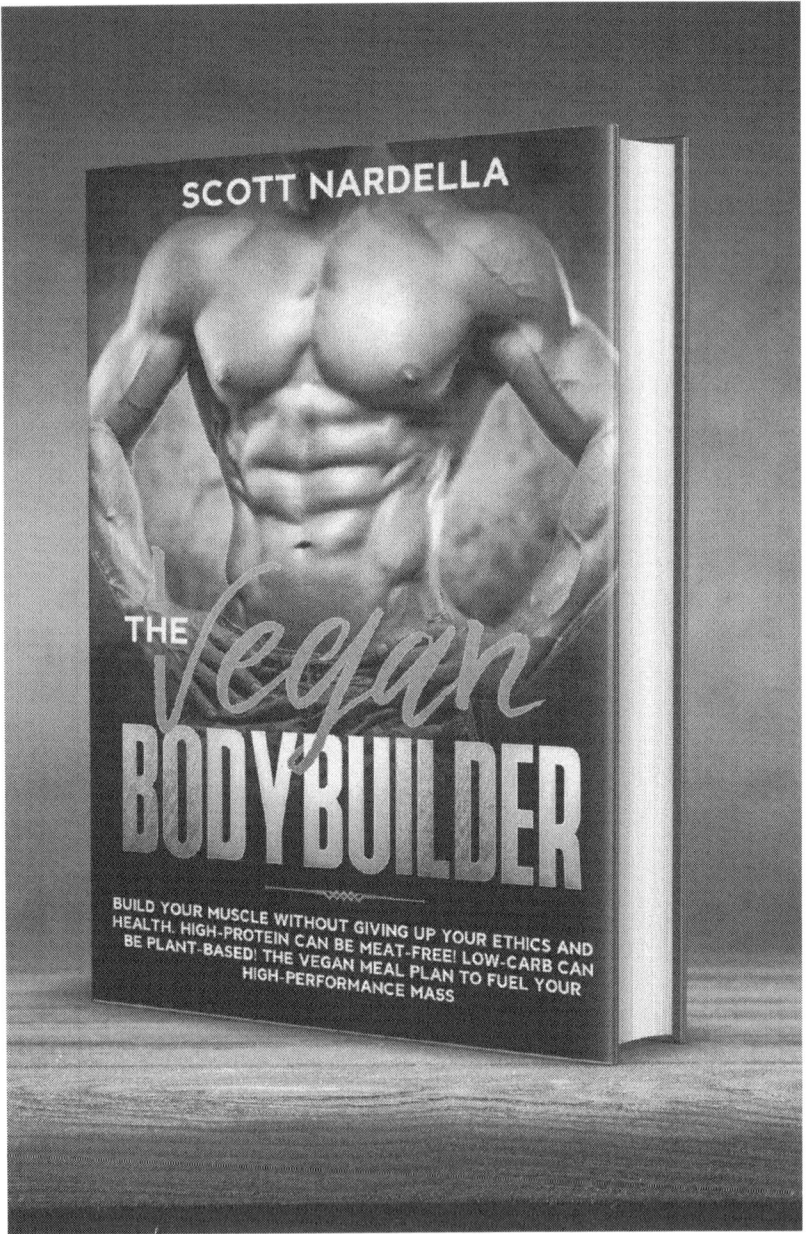

SCOTT NARDELLA

THE *Vegan*
BODYBUILDER

BUILD YOUR MUSCLE WITHOUT GIVING UP YOUR ETHICS AND HEALTH. HIGH-PROTEIN CAN BE MEAT-FREE! LOW-CARB CAN BE PLANT-BASED! THE VEGAN MEAL PLAN TO FUEL YOUR HIGH-PERFORMANCE MASS

Week One

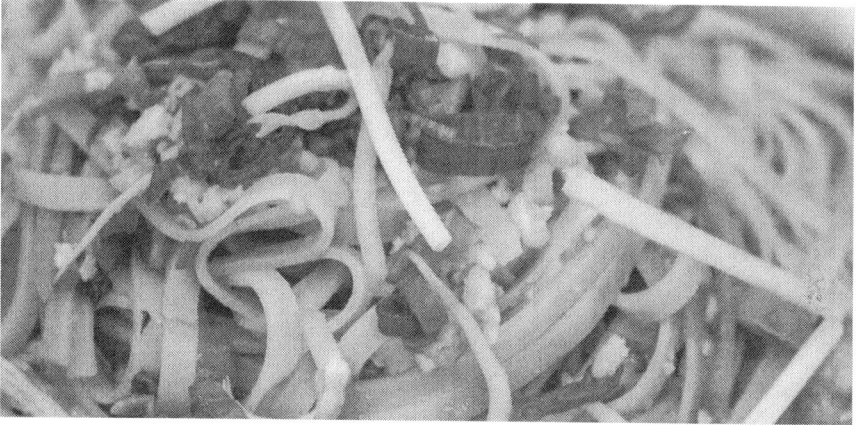

Pad Thai Bowl

Day 1	Breakfast	Pushups Muffins (07)
	Lunch	Boulders Beans Burgers (29)
	Dinner	Chinning Bar Tofu Soup (57)

Day 2	Breakfast	Pumpkin Steel-Cut Oats (02)
	Lunch	Green Pea Risotto (51)
	Dinner	Chickpea Tomato Soup (74)

Day 3	Breakfast	Choco-Quinoa Energy Bowl (03)
	Lunch	Dig Deep Grilled Portobello (53)
	Dinner	Free Weights Split Pea Soup (73)

Day 4	Breakfast	Muesliberry Breakfast (04)
	Lunch	Gear Up Lentils (27)
	Dinner	Beet and Sweet Potato Soup (75)

Day 5	Breakfast	Cinnaspicy Oats (05)
	Lunch	Cauliflower Tacos (28)
	Dinner	Dumbbell Kale Salad (76)

Day 6	Breakfast	French Banana Toast (06)
	Lunch	Chickpeas Gainz Burgers (42)
	Dinner	Coconut and Curry Soup (72)

Day 7	Breakfast	Pushups Muffins (07)
	Lunch	Black Bean Pizza Plate (30)
	Dinner	Creamy Butternut Squash Soup (78)

Week Two

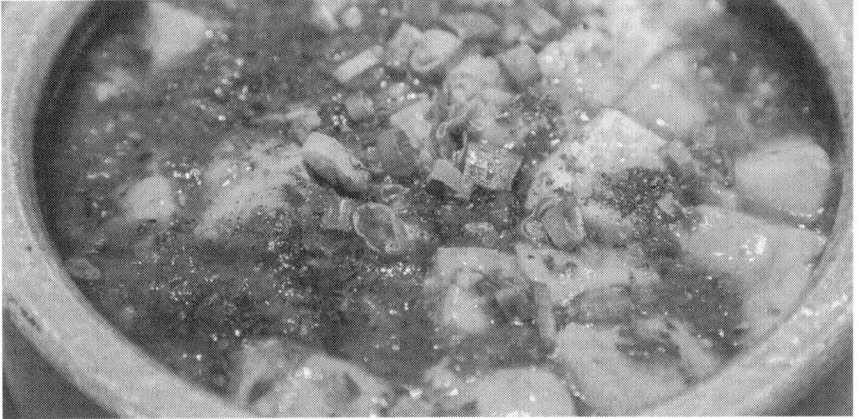

Chin Bar Tofu Soup

Day 8	Breakfast	Vegan Tortilla Breakfast (08)
	Lunch	Under the Bar Burritos (45)
	Dinner	Iron Abs Tabbouleh (55)

Day 9	Breakfast	Leg Day Pancakes (09)
	Lunch	Hulk'n'Bulk Wrap (31)
	Dinner	Mushroom Cream (56)

Day 10	Breakfast	Tropi-Kale Morning Hero (10)
	Lunch	Rice Broccoli Bake (32)
	Dinner	Spicy Root and Lentil Casserole (71)

Day 11	Breakfast	Blueberry Oatmeal Bars (11)
	Lunch	Grain Green and Bean Bowl (33)
	Dinner	Chinning Bar Tofu Soup (57)

Day 12	Breakfast	Quinoa Kettlebell Muffins (12)
	Lunch	Ratatouille (34)
	Dinner	Fast Twitch Quinoa (58)

Day 13	Breakfast	Mexican Beans & Avocado on Toast (25)
	Lunch	Lemon and Thyme Couscous (35)
	Dinner	Miso Noodle Soup (77)

Day 14	Breakfast	Fruit Granola (1)
	Lunch	Quinoa Sushi (36)
	Dinner	Eggplant Parmesan (59)

Week Three

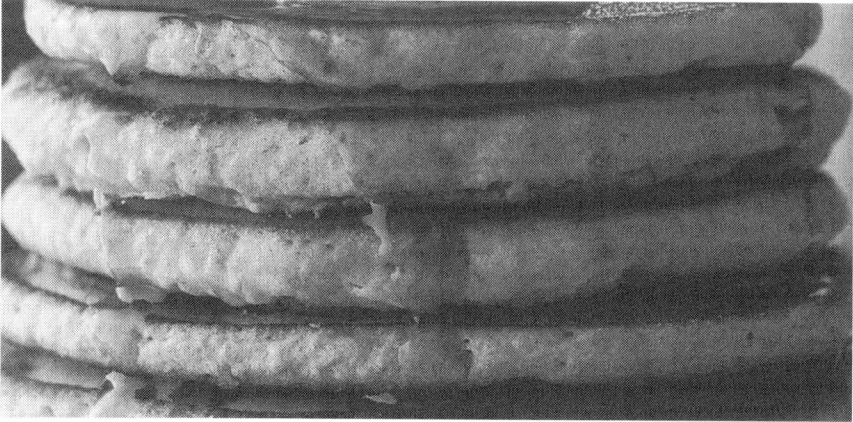

Pumpkin Iron Pancake

Day 15	Breakfast	Vegan Apple Pancakes (24)
	Lunch	Lentil Spinach Curry (37)
	Dinner	Apple-Sunflower Spinach Salad (60)

Day 16	Breakfast	Quinoa Kettlebell Muffins (12)
	Lunch	Gun Show Barley Stew (38)
	Dinner	Tofu Kumquat Radish Salad (80)

Day 17	Breakfast	Pumpkin Iron Pancakes (13)
	Lunch	Power Mushroom Stroganoff (39)
	Dinner	Spaghetti Squash Primavera (61)

Day 18	Breakfast	Quinoa Hercules Bowl (14)
	Lunch	Maxing Out Balsamic Black Beans (40)
	Dinner	Red Peppers and Kale (62)

Day 19	Breakfast	Pull Up Pudding (15)
	Lunch	Rice and Lentils Overload (41)
	Dinner	Clean and Snatch Salad (63)

Day 20	Breakfast	Ten More Reps Parfaits (16)
	Lunch	Boulders Bean Burgers (29)
	Dinner	Caesar Pasta (64)

Day 21	Breakfast	Orange Couscous Boss Breakfast (17)
	Lunch	Pad Thai Bowl (50)
	Dinner	Warm Power Salad (65)

Week Four

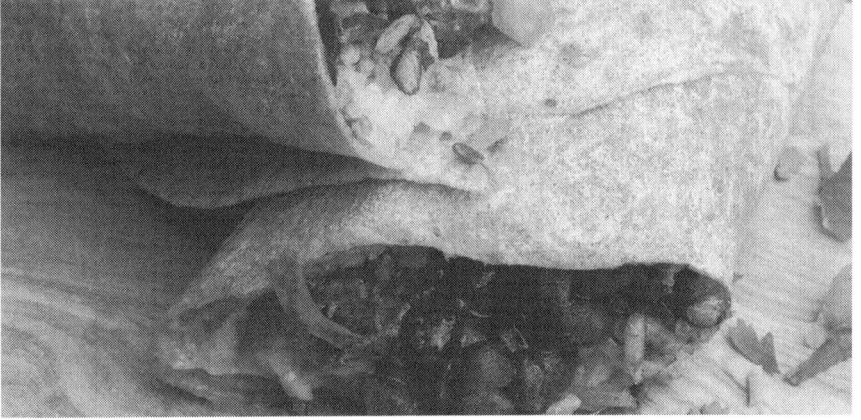

Under the Bar Burritos

Day 22	Breakfast	The Hulk Taco Salad (18)
	Lunch	HIRT Curry Quinoa (43)
	Dinner	Vegan Risotto with Sun Dried Tomatoes (68)

Day 23	Breakfast	Tempeh Miracules Muffin (19)
	Lunch	Split pea soup (44)
	Dinner	Cheese Free mac and cheese (66)

Day 24	Breakfast	Fig and Tofu Oatmeal (20)
	Lunch	Black Bean Pizza Plate (30)
	Dinner	Irish stew (67)

Day 25	Breakfast	Load-it-up! Fajitas (21)
	Lunch	Lentil Soup (54)
	Dinner	Miso Noodle Soup (77)

Day 26	Breakfast	Porridge with Blueberry Compote (23)
	Lunch	Veg Power-Nuggets (46)
	Dinner	Steamed eggplants with peanut dressing (69)

Day 27	Breakfast	Tempeh Miracules Muffin (19)
	Lunch	Crispy Tofu with Hoisin Sauce (48)
	Dinner	Cauliflower Rice Wok (70)

Day 28	Breakfast	No Yeast Cinnamon Rolls (26)
	Lunch	Tofu and Veggies Bulk-Dha-Bowl (47)
	Dinner	Dumbbell Kale Salad (76)

Printed in Great Britain
by Amazon

48901789R00111